THE MARIHUANA PROBLEM

IN THE CITY OF NEW YORK

Sociological, Medical, Psychological
and Pharmacological Studies

by the

MAYOR'S COMMITTEE ON MARIHUANA

THE JAQUES CATTELL PRESS
LANCASTER, PENNSYLVANIA

Printed in U.S.A.

The Livingston Press
Livingston, Columbia County, New York

MAYOR'S COMMITTEE ON MARIHUANA

George B. Wallace, M.D.; *Chairman*

E. H. L. Corwin, Ph.D., *Secretary*

McKeen Cattell, M.D.
Leon H. Cornwall, M.D.
Robert F. Loeb, M.D.
Currier McEwen, M.D.
Bernard S. Oppenheimer, M.D.
Charles Diller Ryan, M.D.

Dudley D. Shoenfeld, M.D.

Ex Officio

Peter F. Amoroso, M.D.
Karl M. Bowman, M.D.
S. S. Goldwater, M.D.
John L. Rice, M.D.

Special Advisers for Clinical Study

Karl M. Bowman, M.D.
David Wechsler, Ph.D.

Supervisors of Clinical Study

J. Murray Steele, M.D.
S. Bernard Wortis, M.D.

Table of Contents

Foreword by the Honorable F. H. La Guardia,
Mayor of the City of New York

Foreword

As Mayor of the City of New York, it is my duty to foresee and take steps to prevent the development of hazards to the health, safety, and welfare of our citizens. When rumors were recently circulated concerning the smoking of marihuana by large segments of our population and even by school children, I sought advice from The New York Academy of Medicine, as is my custom when confronted with problems of medical import. On the Academy's recommendation I appointed a special committee to make a thorough sociological and scientific investigation, and secured funds from three Foundations with which to finance these studies.

My own interest in marihuana goes back many years, to the time when I was a member of the House of Representatives and, in that capacity, heard of the use of marihuana by soldiers stationed in Panama. I was impressed at that time with the report of an Army Board of Inquiry which emphasized the relative harmlessness of the drug and the fact that it played a very little role, if any, in problems of delinquency and crime in the Canal Zone.

The report of the present investigations covers every phase of the problem and is of practical value not only to our own city but to communities throughout the country. It is a basic contribution to medicine and pharmacology.

I am glad that the sociological, psychological, and medical ills commonly attributed to marihuana have been found to be exaggerated insofar as the City of New York is concerned. I hasten to point out, however, that the findings are to be interpreted only as a reassuring report of progress and not as encouragement to indulgence, for I shall continue to enforce the laws prohibiting the use of marihuana until and if complete findings may justify an amendment to existing laws. The scientific part of the research will be continued in the hope that the drug may prove to possess therapeutic value for the control of drug addiction.

I take this occasion to express my appreciation and gratitude to the members of my committee, to The New York Academy of Medicine, and to the Commonwealth Fund, the Friedam Foundation, and the New York Foundation which supportd these important investigations so generously.

F. H. LaGuardia
Mayor

Foreword

As Mayor of the City of New York, it is my duty to foresee and take steps to prevent the development of hazards to the health, safety, and welfare of our citizens. When rumors were recently circulated concerning the smoking of marihuana by large segments of our population and even by school children, I sought advice from The New York Academy of Medicine, as is my custom when confronted with problems of medical nature. On the Academy's recommendation I appointed a special committee to make a thorough sociological and scientific investigation, and secured funds from three foundations with which to finance these studies.

[illegible]

I take this occasion to express my appreciation and gratitude to the members of my committee, to The New York Academy of Medicine, and to the Commonwealth Fund, the Friedsam Foundation and the New York Foundation which supported these important investigations so generously.

F. H. La Guardia
Mayor

Introduction

E. H. L. Corwin, Ph.D., Secretary

On September 13, 1938, The New York Academy of Medicine was informed of Mayor LaGuardia's concern about the marihuana problem and of his desire "that some impartial body such as The New York Academy of Medicine make a survey of existing knowledge on this subject and carry out any observations required to determine the pertinent facts regarding this form of drug addiction and the necessity for its control." The Mayor's request was referred to the Committee on Public Health Relations of the Academy, which Committee on October 17, 1938 authorized the appointment of a special subcommittee to study the Mayor's request.

This Subcommittee, consisting of Dr. George B. Wallace, Chairman, Dr. E. H. L. Corwin, Secretary, and Drs. McKeen Cattell, Leon H. Cornwall, Robert F. Loeb, Currier McEwen, B. S. Oppenheimer, Charles Diller Ryan, and Dudley D. Shoenfeld, reviewed the existing literature on the subject. On the basis of this review, the Subcommittee could come to no conclusion regarding the effect of marihuana upon the psychological and physiological functions of the human being. Nor were attempts to learn the extent of the use of marihuana in New York City any more successful. A conference with representatives of the Police Department, the Department of Education, the Department of Correction, the Psychiatric Division of the Department of Hospitals, the Court of Domestic Relations, the District Attorney's office, and the Citizens Committee on the Control of Crime served to emphasize the existing differences of opinion regarding the extent of the use of marihuana in this city and its relationship to crime.

The Subcommittee therefore came to the conclusion that, in view of the possibility that marihuana smoking might constitute an important social problem, it was time that a study of its effects be made based upon well-established evidence, and prepared an outline of methods of procedure for the study of the problem. It recommended that such a study should be divided into two parts: (1) a sociological study dealing with the extent of marihuana smoking and the methods by which the drug is obtained; in what districts and among what races, classes or types of persons the use is most prevalent; whether certain social conditions are factors in its use;

and what relation there is between its use and criminal or anti-social acts; and (2) a clinical study to determine by means of controlled experiments the physiological and psychological effects of marihuana on different types of persons; the question as to whether it causes physical or mental deterioration; and its possible therapeutic effects in the treatment of disease or of other drug addictions.

The Committee on Public Health Relations adopted the report of its Subcommittee and recommended to Mayor LaGuardia that he appoint a special committee to carry out the proposed study. Accordingly in January, 1939, he appointed the Mayor's Committee on Marihuana, composed of the members of the Subcommittee of the Committee on Public Health Relations which recommended the study and four ex-officio members: Dr. Peter F. Amoroso, First Deputy Commissioner (later Commissioner) of Correction; Dr. Karl M. Bowman, Director of the Psychiatric Division of the Department of Hospitals; Dr. S. S. Goldwater, Commissioner of Hospitals; and Dr. John L. Rice, Commissioner of Health. Upon his accession to the commissionership of the Department of Hospitals, Dr. Willard C. Rappleye succeeded Dr. Goldwater as a member of this Committee.

This Committee studied the broad outlines of the proposed plans for about a year before work was actually begun. At its first meeting in March 1939 two subcommittees were appointed: one, consisting of Drs. Shoenfeld, Ryan, and Corwin to plan the sociological study, and the other, composed of Drs. Cattell, Bowman, Cornwall, and Loeb to work out the details of the clinical study. Drs. Bowman and Wechsler were appointed as special advisers for the clinical study and Dr. J. Murray Steele and Dr. S. Bernard Wortis as the supervisors of this study.

The studies were made possible by the financial support of three Foundations, the Friedsam Foundation, the New York Foundation, and the Commonwealth Fund, each of which donated $7,500. The whole amounts granted by the Friedsam Foundation and the Commonwealth Fund and $5,000 of the New York Foundation's grant were to be applied to the clinical study; the remaining $2,500 given by the New York Foundation was earmarked for the sociological study. The Research Council of the Department of Hospitals undertook the financial supervision of the clinical study and The New York Academy of Medicine that of the sociological study.

The sociological study proceeded under the active direction of Dr. Dudley D. Shoenfeld and was carried out by six police officers who were trained by Dr. Shoenfeld as social investigators. In acknowledgment of the great help rendered to the Committee by these officers, the Committee passed the following resolution at its meeting on March 18, 1941.

"Now that the sociological study of the marihuana problem in New York City has been completed, the Mayor's Committee on Marihuana wishes to record its appreciation of the Mayor's interest in this problem and his placing at the disposal of the Committee the services of the Narcotic Squad Division of the Police Department.

"Without the cooperation of Commissioner Valentine, Inspector Curtayne, Lieutenant Cooper, Sergeant Boylan, and Detective Loures, this study would have been impossible. They helped in planning it and assigned to the Committee six members of the Force, four men and two women, whose intelligence, interest in the work, and desire to obtain the facts of the situation were of invaluable aid in obtaining the information on which the sociological report is based. The four men and two women assigned to us made painstaking observations and reports, acted as investigators and social workers and not as police officers, and brought to the performance of this task a native intelligence, specialized training, and civic interest. The thanks of the Committee are due to them and through them to their superiors."

The clinical study consisted of two parts,—the medical, including psychiatric, and the psychological. Dr. Karl M. Bowman directed the medical and psychiatric part of this study and Dr. David Wechsler the psychological part. The members of the Committee closely supervised the work during the course of the study. The staff of the clinical study included:

Samuel Allentuck, M.D., Psychiatrist, who was in charge.

Louis Gitzelter, M.D.
Frank Anker, M.D. } Assistant Physicians

Robert S. Morrow, Ph.D.
Florence Halpern, M.A.
Adolph G. Woltmann, M.A. } Psychologists

Miss Rose Horowitz who was the secretary-stenographer and bookkeeper.

The Committee is indebted to the Department of Hospitals for making available two small wards and office space in the Welfare Hospital (now known as the Goldwater Memorial Hospital), to Dr. Chrisman G. Scherf, the Superintendent of the hospital, and to the laboratory staff of the Third Medical Division for their assistance in the conduct of laboratory experiments. Acknowledgment should also be made of the services of Dr. Robert C. Batterman who interpreted the electrocardiograms and Dr. Hans Strauss for the electroence phalographic work. Professor Walter R. Miles of Yale University assisted in the planning of the psychological part of the study.

This whole undertaking would have been impossible without the help and cooperation of Dr. Peter F. Amoroso, of the Department of Correction, who, aside from his services as a member of the Committee, was responsible for arrangements for volunteers from among the prisoners at the Riker's Island Penitentiary. Thanks are due also to the entire medical staff of the Riker's Island Hospital for their assistance in the narcotic addiction study.

At the suggestion of Dr. Cattell a pharmacological study was done in the Department of Pharmacology of Cornell Medical School by Dr. S. Loewe. Dr. W. Modell collaborated in this work. We are indebted to Dr. Roger Adams, Professor of Chemistry at the University of Illinois, and to Dr. H. J. Wollner, Consulting Chemist of the United States Treasury Department, who supplied some of the active principles of marihuana which were used in the study.

The names of those who conducted the investigations are given under the different chapters. Those sections of the report for which no author is indicated have been written by the Chairman of the Committee.

The tremendous task of compiling, editing, and revising the reports was undertaken by Dr. George B. Wallace, the Chairman of the Committee, and Miss Elizabeth V. Cunningham of the staff of the Committee on Public Health Relations of The New York Academy of Medicine. They had the assistance of Dr. Dudley D. Shoenfeld who prepared the sociological report, Dr. David Wechsler who revised the psychological reports, and Dr. McKeen Cattell who edited the pharmacological report.

In the judgment of the Committee, this painstaking study should be of considerable value from a scientific and social viewpoint.

THE SOCIOLOGICAL STUDY

DUDLEY D. SHOENFELD, M.D.

Introduction

In order to understand fully the purpose and scope of this particular part of the survey conducted by the Mayor's Committee on Marihuana, a brief digest of the history of the growth and usage of this drug is essential.

Indian hemp, from which marihuana (the American synonym for hashish) is obtained, has been known to man for more than three thousand years. This plant, although originally indigenous to Central Asia, is now found in practically every section of the world, growing either wild or cultivated, legally or illegally.

When originally discovered, the use to which this plant was principally put was the conversion of its fiber for commercial purposes in the production of cord, twine and textiles. Shortly thereafter its pharmaceutical properties were employed in the practice of medicine and surgery. Authoritative proof is available that the Chinese found it valuable as an effective anesthetic in surgery as far back as two thousand years. It was not until approximately the tenth century that the peoples of Africa and Asia began to use it in a rather indiscriminate manner for its intoxicating effects.

Very shortly after its usage became popular, this drug engaged the attention of the various African and Asian governments, as well as of lay persons interested in medical, religious and sociological problems. Some of these very early investigators propounded the theory that physical and mental deterioration was the direct result of smoking hashish. Others extolled its benefits, deeming it actually essential to life, and urged people to indulge in it.

During this early period, the peoples of Europe were aware of the use of hashish in Africa and Asia, and considered it a vice particularly common to the peoples of those continents. In the nineteenth century their interest was raised to a high pitch because of the fictional reports of the smoking of hashish given by the romanticists of that period.

These individuals, who had the power of the pen, experimentally indulged in the smoking of hashish, and described in an expansive, subjective manner the effects the drug had upon them. A review of the fanciful literature reveals that in most instances these writings referred to the authors' experiences with toxic doses. Summed up, the conclusions were that hashish could cause psychotic episodes and even death and that prolonged use would result in physical and mental deterioration. The exalted position held by these romanticists tended to influence the Europeans to accept their conclusions as scientific monographs on the subject of hashish, so that the smoking of hashish did not become popular with them. However, in recent years there has been a fairly wide participation on the part of Europeans in smoking hashish or marihuana, but it is referred to as an American vice. This allows one to infer that whereas the knowledge pertaining to this habit was very early recognized in Europe, at the present time participation in it is from their point of view the direct result of its introduction into Europe not from Africa and Asia, but from America.

In America, Indian hemp was planted in the New England colonies, solely for commercial purposes, as early as the seventeenth century. At the present time it can be found growing either wild or cultivated, legally or illegally, in practically all our States. Lawful cultivation is confined principally to the states of Kentucky, Illinois, Minnesota and Wisconsin. It has been estimated that not more than ten thousand acres are devoted to its legal production. It is of value commercially in the manufacture of rope, twine and textiles. The seed is used for bird-food, and the oil extracted from the seed is occasionally used as a substitute for linseed oil in the preparation of artists' paints. A rosin extracted from the plant is used in the production of pharmaceutical preparations.

Since the history of hemp cultivation in America dates back to the seventeenth century, it is exceedingly interesting, but difficult to explain, that the smoking of marihuana did not become a problem in our country until approximately twenty years ago, and that it has become an acute problem associated with a great deal of publicity only in the past ten years.

The origin of the word marihuana is in doubt. Some authorities are of the opinion that it is derived from the Portuguese word "mariguano" meaning intoxicant. Others are of the opinion that it has its derivation in the Mexican words for "Mary and Jane." The introduction into the United States of the practice of smoking marihuana has been the subject of a great deal of speculation. The most tenable hypothesis at the present time is that it was introduced by Mexicans entering our country.

It is accepted that in Mexico marihuana smoking is an old, established practice. Therefore, it would appear logical to assume that Mexican laborers crossing our border into the Southwest carried this practice with them. Having used marihuana in their native land, they found it natural to continue smoking it in the new country, and planted it for personal consumption. Once available, it was soon made use of by our citizens. At the present time, the smoking of marihuana is widespread in this nation.

Believing that marihuana smoking might be deleterious, and knowing it to be widespread, federal and municipal governments, private individuals, and such agencies as the Opium Advisory Association, the International Narcotic Education Association and others investigated the subject. These investigative organizations have contributed a great deal of data and pertinent information to the knowledge of the use of marihuana.

The mass of information so obtained when untangled can be summed up with the general statement that a majority of investigators are of the opinion that marihuana smoking is deleterious, although a minority maintain that it is innocuous. The majority believe that marihuana smoking is widespread among school children; that the dispensers of the drug are organized to such an extent that they encourage the use of marihuana in order to create an ever-increasing market; that juvenile delinquency is directly related to the effects of the drug; that it is a causative factor in a large percentage of our major crimes and sexual offenses; and that physical and mental deterioration are the direct result of the prolonged habit of smoking marihuana.

As a result of these official and semi-official conclusions in regard to the disastrous effects produced by this habit, the newspapers and magazines of our country have given it wide publicity. At this point it may be profitable to give the conclusions of some of the investigators and quote the publicity associated with it.

In a pamphlet "Marihuana or Indian Hemp and Its Preparations" issued by the International Narcotic Education Association, one finds:

"Marihuana is a most virile and powerful stimulant. The physiological effect of this drug produces a peculiar psychic exaltation and derangement of the central nervous system. The stage of exaltation and confusion, more marked in some addicts than in others is generally followed by a stage of depression.

"Sometimes the subject passes into a semi-conscious state, experiencing vivid and extravagant dreams which vary according to the individual character and mentality. In some the stage is one of self-satisfaction and well-being. In others, it is alarming, presenting the fear of some imminent and indefinite danger or of impending death. Later the dreams are sometimes followed by a state of complete unconsciousness. Sometimes convulsive attacks and acute mania are developed.

"The narcotic content in marihuana decreases the rate of heart beat and causes irregularity of the pulse. Death may result from the effect upon the heart.

"Prolonged use of marihuana frequently develops a delirious rage which sometimes leads to high crimes, such as assault and murder. Hence marihuana has been called the 'killer drug.' The habitual use of this narcotic poison always causes a very marked mental deterioration and sometimes produces insanity. Hence marihuana is frequently called 'loco weed.' (Loco is the Spanish word for crazy.)

"While the marihuana habit leads to physical wreckage and mental decay, its effects upon character and morality are even more devastating. The victim frequently undergoes such degeneracy that he will lie and steal without scruple; he becomes utterly untrustworthy and often drifts into the underworld where, with his degenerate companions, he commits high crimes and misdemeanors. Marihuana sometimes gives man the lust to kill unreasonably and without motive. Many cases of assault, rape, robbery and murder are traced to the use of marihuana."[1]

In an article published in the New York Daily Worker, New York, Saturday, December 28th, 1940, there appeared under the column headed "HEALTH ADVICE":

"A DRUG AND INSANITY.

"Bill Wilson was strolling by his favorite soda joint on the way home from high school when he heard a familiar voice whisper loudly, 'Hey, Bill, c'mere!' Behind the Texaco billboard, he found his side-kick Jim, who said excitedly, 'I got some reefers!' 'Reefers, What're they?' Mysteriously, Jim reached into his pocket and pulled out two large cigarettes. 'Marihuana!' Jim's pupils dilated. 'Come on over to the club and we'll smoke 'em. Boy, that's fun!'

"Bill is only one of thousands of new marihuana smokers created yearly among boys and girls of high school age. What is this drug? It is a narcotic in the same class as opium and is derived from a plant, which grows wild, extensively in some parts. For this reason, it is hard to control and the drug is easy to obtain at very little cost.

---

(1) International Narcotic Education Association. Marihuana or Indiana Hemp and Its Preparations. Los Angeles, 1936.

"Smoking of the weed is habit-forming. It destroys the will-power, releases restraints, and promotes insane reactions. Continued use causes the face to become bloated, the eyes bloodshot, the limbs weak and trembling, and the mind sinks into insanity. Robberies, thrill murders, sex crimes and other offenses result.

"When the habit is first started, the symptoms are milder, yet powerful enough. The smoker loses all sense of time and space so that he can't judge distances, he loses his self-control, and his imagination receives considerable stimulation.

"The habit can be cured only by the most severe methods. The addict must be put into an institution, where the drug is gradually withdrawn, his general health is built up, and he is kept there until he has enough will-power to withstand the temptation to again take to the weed.

"The spread of this terrible fad can be stopped only when the unscrupulous criminals trafficking in the drug are rooted out."

Dr. Robert P. Walton, Professor of Pharmacology of the School of Medicine of the University of Mississippi, has written a most comprehensive book on the subject of marihuana, embodying in detail pharmacological and social studies.(1) A chapter on the "Present Status of the Marihuana Vice in the United States" was prepared by Dr. Frank R. Gomila, Commissioner of Public Safety of New Orleans, and Madeline C. G. Lambou, Assistant City Chemist. They refer to New Orleans as being possibly the first large city in the United States where the drug habit became widely established among the native population, and they therefore believe that the authorities in this city had a decided opportunity to observe the progress of the smoking of marihuana as a social problem. Referring specifically to the use of marihuana among school children, they state that reporters in New Orleans not only heard about but observed large numbers of boys of school age actually buying and smoking marihuana cigarettes. One peddler was so brazen as to keep his stock under the street stairs to a girls' high school.

Inquiries further revealed that school children of forty-four schools in New Orleans (only a few of these were high schools) smoked marihuana. As a result of exposure and widespread agitation, "Verifications came in by the hundreds from harassed parents, teachers, neighborhood pastors, priests, welfare workers and club women. Warrington House for boys was full of children who had become habituated to the use of cannabis. The superintendent of

(1) Walton, R. P. Marihuana: America's New Drug Problem. J. B. Lippincott Co., Philadelphia, 1938.

the Children's Bureau reported that there were many problem children there who had come under the influence and two who had run away because they couldn't get their 'muggles' at the Bureau. The Director of Kingsley House for boys received many pleas from fathers of boys who had come under the influence and were charged with petty crimes. After personally seeing these boys in an hysterical condition or on the well-known 'laughing jags,' the director termed the situation decidedly grave. The Waif's Home, at this time, was reputedly full of children, both white and colored, who had been brought in under the influence of the drug. Marihuana cigarettes could be bought almost as readily as sandwiches. Their cost was two for a quarter. The children solved the problem of cost by pooling pennies among the members of a group and then passing the cigarettes from one to another, all the puffs being carefully counted. . . .

"The result of these investigations ended in a wholesale arrest of more than 150 persons. Approximately one hundred underworld dives, soft-drink establishments, night clubs, grocery stores, and private homes were searched in the police raid. Addicts, hardened criminals, gangsters, women of the streets, sailors of all nationalities, bootleggers, boys and girls—many flashily dressed in silks and furs, others in working clothes—all were rounded up in the net which Captain Smith and his squad had set.

". . . Notwithstanding the thoroughness with which this police roundup was carried out, it did not entirely eradicate in one stroke a vice which had already become so well-established. During the next few years New Orleans experienced a crime wave which unquestionably was greatly aggravated by the influence of this drug habit. Payroll and bank guards were doubled, but this did not prevent some of the most spectacular hold-ups in the history of the city. Youngsters known to be 'muggle-heads' fortified themselves with the narcotic and proceeded to shoot down police, bank clerks and casual by-standers. Mr. Eugene Stanley, at that time District Attorney, declared that many of the crimes in New Orleans and the South were thus committed by criminals who relied on the drug to give them a false courage and freedom from restraint. Dr. George Roeling, Coroner, reported that of 450 prisoners investigated, 125 were confirmed users of marihuana. Dr. W. B. Graham, State Narcotic Officer, declared in 1936 that 60 per cent of the crimes committed in New Orleans were by marihuana users."(1)

The Mayor's Committee on Marihuana decided to confine its investigations to a limited area. For a number of reasons the Borough of Manhattan seemed to be the most profitable section of the city in which to concentrate. In order to crystallize our particular project we deemed it advisable to direct our efforts to finding answers to the following questions:

1. To what extent is marihuana used?
2. What is the method of retail distribution?
3. What is the general attitude of the marihuana smoker toward society and toward the use of the drug?
4. What is the relationship between marihuana and eroticism?
5. What is the relationship between marihuana and crime?
6. What is the relationship between marihuana and juvenile delinquency?

In the course of our investigations, we have made extensive use of subjective data obtained from those who were actual smokers of marihuana and directly acquainted with its effects and those who were not smokers, but, because of residence, occupation or other interests, were acquainted with the general subject.

Organization of Staff

In October, 1939, Police Commissioner Lewis J. Valentine designated Deputy Chief Inspector Daniel Curtayne, Lieutenant Edward Cooper, Sergeant Bernard Boylan and Detective Joseph Loures of the Narcotic Squad of the Police Department of the City of New York to cooperate with the Mayor's Committee on Marihuana. These police officials submitted a list of intelligent young officers with a suitable background. From this list, six officers were selected: two policewomen, and four policemen, one of whom was a Negro. They were: Mr. James Coen, Mr. William Connolly, Mr. Benjamin Weissner, Mr. John Hughes, Miss Adelaide Knowles and Miss Olive Cregan. These police officers were encouraged to read literature on the subject of marihuana and to familiarize themselves with some of the characteristics of the plant, as well as of

(1) Walton, R. P. Marihuana: America's New Drug Problem. J. B. Lippincott Co., Philadelphia, 1938.

marihuana cigarettes. They became expert in detecting the aroma of burning marihuana, and were thus able to recognize it and to identify its use in a social gathering.

Regular assignments were made by the director of the survey. At intervals each officer dictated a general report on his activities and findings to a stenographer engaged by the Committee. Frequent conferences were held in the office of the director of the survey, at which time individual reports were discussed in detail and evaluated. An attempt was made to give the "marihuana squad" a psychological approach to the performance of their duties.

At no time were these officers permitted to make known their activity to other members of the police force, or to make arrests. This arrangement was considered essential in order that they might maintain an effective role of investigator without being in any respect recognized as police officers. Although they were members of the police force and constantly in contact with violators of law, their immediate superiors cooperated to an extreme degree by allowing the "marihuana squad" to report directly to the director of the survey.

While on duty the squad actually "lived" in the environment in which marihuana smoking or peddling was suspected. They frequented poolrooms, bars and grills, dime-a-dance halls, other dance halls to which they took their own partners, theatres—backstage and in the audience—roller-skating rinks, subways, public toilets, parks and docks. They consorted with the habitués of these places, chance acquaintances on the street, loiterers around schools, subways and bus terminals. They posed as "suckers" from out of town and as students in colleges and high schools.

We highly commend these officers individually for their exceptionally good performances. The aid given by Deputy Chief Inspector Daniel Curtayne, Lieutenant Edward Cooper, Sergeant Bernard Boylan and Detective Joseph Loures throughout deserves special mention and appreciation. At times we must have been a source of annoyance to them, but our requests were always cheerfully met and assistance heartily extended.

Method of Retail Distribution

In general, marihuana is used in the form of a cigarette. Occasionally some individuals chew the "weed" and seem to get the

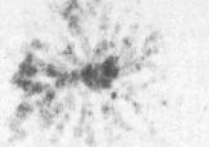

same effect as do others through smoking. The common names for the cigarette are: muggles, reefers, Indian hemp, weed, tea, gage and sticks. Cigarettes made of marihuana differ in size as do cigarettes made of tobacco: they are long, short, thick or thin.

The price varies in accordance with the accepted opinion as to the potency of the marihuana used in the cigarettes, and this appears to be determined by the place of origin. The cheapest brand is known as "sass-fras," and retails for approximately three for 50 cents. It is made of the marihuana that is grown in the United States. Smokers do not consider such marihuana very potent. They have found that they must consume a greater number of cigarettes in order to obtain the desired effect colloquially termed as "high." This opinion, expressed by smokers in the Borough of Manhattan, is at variance with that of some authorities who believe that marihuana grown in the United States is as potent as the marihuana grown in other countries.

The "panatella" cigarette, occasionally referred to as "meserole," is considered to be more potent than the "sass-fras" and usually retails for approximately 25 cents each. The hemp from which the "panatella" is made comes from Central and South America.

"Gungeon" is considered by the marihuana smoker as the highest grade of marihuana. It retails for about one dollar per cigarette. The "kick" resulting from the use of this cigarette is reached more quickly than from the use of "sass-fras" or "panatella." It appears to be the consensus that the marihuana used to make the "gungeon" comes from Africa. The sale of this cigarette is restricted to a clientele whose economic status is of a higher level than the majority of marihuana smokers.

A confirmed marihuana user can readily distinguish the quality and potency of various brands, just as the habitual cigarette or cigar smoker is able to differentiate between the qualities of tobacco. Foreign-made cigarette paper is often used in order to convince the buyer that the "tea is right from the boat."

There are two channels for the distribution of marihuana cigarettes—the independent peddler and the "tea-pad." From general observations, conversations with "pad" owners, and discussions with peddlers, the investigators estimated that there were about 500 "tea-pads" in Harlem and at least 500 peddlers.

A "tea-pad" is a room or an apartment in which people gather to smoke marihuana. The majority of such places are located in the Harlem district. It is our impression that the landlord, the agent, the superintendent or the janitor is aware of the purposes for which the premises are rented.

The "tea-pad" is furnished according to the clientele it expects to serve. Usually, each "tea-pad" has comfortable furniture, a radio, victrola or, as in most instances, a rented nickelodeon. The lighting is more or less uniformly dim, with blue predominating. An incense burner is considered part of the furnishings. The walls are frequently decorated with pictures of nude subjects suggestive of perverted sexual practices. The furnishings, as described, are believed to be essential as a setting for those participating in smoking marihuana.

Most "tea-pads" have their trade restricted to the sale of marihuana. Some places did sell marihuana and whisky, and a few places also served as houses of prostitution. Only one "tea-pad" was found which served as a house of prostitution, and in which one could buy marihuana, whisky and opium.

The marihuana smoker derives greater satisfaction if he is smoking in the presence of others. His attitude in the "tea-pad" is that of a relaxed individual, free from the anxieties and cares of the realities of life. The "tea-pad" takes on the atmosphere of a very congenial social club. The smoker readily engages in conversation with strangers, discussing freely his pleasant reactions to the drug and philosophizing on subjects pertaining to life in a manner which, at times, appears to be out of keeping with his intellectual level. A constant observation was the extreme willingness to share and puff on each other's cigarettes. A boisterous, rowdy atmosphere did not prevail and on the rare occasions when there appeared signs indicative of a belligerent attitude on the part of a smoker, he was ejected or forced to become more tolerant and quiescent. One of the most interesting setups of a "tea-pad," which was clearly not along orthodox lines from the business point of view, was a series of pup tents arranged on a roof-top in Harlem. Those present proceeded to smoke their cigarettes in the tents. When the desired effect of the drug had been obtained they all emerged into the open and engaged in a discussion of their admiration of the stars and beauties of nature.

Because of the possibility of spreading disease, note should be taken of what seems to be a custom known as "pick-up" smoking. It is an established practice whereby a marihuana cigarette is lit and

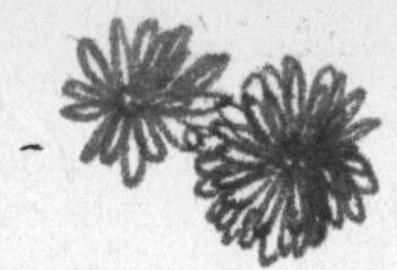

after one or two inhalations is passed on to the next person. This procedure is repeated until all present have had an opportunity to take a puff or two on the cigarette.

Occasionally a "tea-pad" owner may have peddlers who sell their wares in other localities and at the same time serve as procurers for those who wish to smoke marihuana on the premises.

One also finds other methods of retail distribution. After proper introduction, one may be able to purchase the cigarette in certain places. This is not an easy procedure, but it can be accomplished. In some "bar and grill" 's, restaurants and bars our investigators were able to establish contact with someone who, in turn, would introduce them to a peddler who apparently made regular rounds of these places in order to sell cigarettes. It appears that the owners of such places are not aware of this practice, and in many instances they would discharge any employee known to be directly or indirectly associated with the sale of marihuana.

On rare occasions public guides, if properly approached, would refer one to a place where the "reefer" could be bought. There was no evidence that the guide received money when acting as go-between. Terminal porters, mainly Negroes, appeared to be more directly connected with the traffic of marihuana. They were more conversant with the subject and it was easier for them to establish contact between purchaser and peddler.

Marihuana smoking is very common in the theatres of Harlem according to the observations of the investigators. We have reason to believe that in some instances, perhaps few in number, employees actually sold cigarettes on the premises. In the Harlem dance halls smoking was frequently observed either in the lavatories or on the main floor. The patrons as well as the musicians were seen in the act of smoking. There was no evidence of sales being made by employees on the premises, or that there was any gain on the part of the owners or employees in permitting this practice. Whereas the smoking of marihuana was not encouraged, nothing was done to prohibit such practice.

There are specific sections in the Borough of Manhattan where the sale of marihuana cigarettes appears to be localized: 1) the Harlem district; 2) the Broadway area, a little east and west of Broadway and extending from 42nd Street to 59th Street. While it is true that one may buy the cigarette in other districts, it is not as easily obtainable as in the two localities mentioned.

The Mental Attitude of the Marihuana Smoker Toward Society and Marihuana

Most of the smokers of marihuana coming within the scope of our survey were unemployed, and of the others most had part-time employment.

Occasional, as well as confirmed, users were all aware of the laws pertaining to the illegal use of the drug. They did not indulge in its use with a spirit of braggadocio or as a challenge to law as has been reported by some investigators in other districts. They did not express remorse concerning their use of marihuana, nor did they blame this habit as a causative factor in the production of special difficulties in their personal lives. Except for musicians there appeared to be no attempt at secretiveness on the part of the habitual smoker. This attitude is in marked contrast to that usually taken by those addicted to morphine, cocaine, or heroin.

The consensus of marihuana users is that the drug is not harmful and that infrequent or constant use of marihuana does not result in physical or mental deterioration.

In describing the most common reaction to the drug they always stated that it made them feel "high." Elaboration of just what the smoker meant by "high" varied with the individual. However, there was common agreement that a feeling of adequacy and efficiency was induced by the use of marihuana and that current mental conflicts were allayed. Organic illness was not given as a cause for smoking "reefers."

A person may be a confirmed smoker for a prolonged period, and give up the drug voluntarily without experiencing any craving for it or exhibiting withdrawal symptoms. He may, at some time later on, go back to its use. Others may remain infrequent users of the cigarette, taking one or two a week, or only when the "social setting" calls for participation. From time to time we had one of our investigators associate with a marihuana user. The investigator would bring up the subject of smoking. This would invariably lead to the suggestion that they obtain some marihuana cigarettes. They would seek a "tea-pad," and if it was closed the smoker and our investigator would calmly resume their previous activity, such as, the discussion of life in general or the playing of pool. There were apparently no signs indicative of frustration in the smoker at not being able to gratify the desire for the drug. We consider this point highly significant since it is so contrary to the experience of users of other narcotics. A similar situation occurring in one addicted to the use of morphine, cocaine or heroin would result in a compulsive attitude on the part of the addict to obtain the drug. If unable to secure it, there would be obvious physical and mental manifestations of frustration. This may be considered presumptive evidence that there is no true addiction in the medical sense associated with the use of marihuana.

The confirmed marihuana smoker consumes perhaps from six to ten cigarettes per day. He appears to be quite conscious of the quantity he requires to reach the effect called "high." Once the desired effect is obtained he cannot be persuaded to consume more. He knows when he has had enough. The smoker determines for himself the point of being "high," and is ever-conscious of preventing himself from becoming "too high." This fear of being "too high" must be associated with some form of anxiety which causes the smoker, should he accidentally reach that point, immediately to institute measures so that he can "come down." It has been found that the use of beverages such as beer, or a sweet soda pop, is an effective measure. Smokers insist that "it does something to the stomach" and that it is always associated with "belching." A cold shower will also have the effect of bringing the person "down."

Smokers have repeatedly stated that the consumption of whisky while smoking negates the potency of the drug. They find it is very difficult to get "high" while drinking whisky, and because of that smokers will not drink whisky while using the "weed." They do, however, consume large quantities of sweet wines. It is their contention that this mild alcoholic beverage aids the drug in producing the desired effect. Most marihuana smokers insist that the appetite is increased as the result of smoking.

We have been unable to confirm the opinion expressed by some investigators that marihuana smoking is the first step in the use of such drugs as cocaine, morphine and heroin. The instances are extremely rare where the habit of marihuana smoking is associated with addiction to these other narcotics.

Marihuana and Eroticism

In the popular agitation against the use of marihuana, its erotic effects have been stressed repeatedly. As previously stated in this report, our investigators visited many "tea-pads" in the Borough of Manhattan. It is true that lewd pictures decorated the walls but they did not find that they were attracting attention or comment among the clientele. In fact one of the investigators who was concentrating his attention on the relation between marihuana and eroticism stated in his report that he found himself embarrassed in that he was the only one who examined the pictures on the wall.

Numerous conversations with smokers of marihuana revealed only occasional instances in which there was any relation between the drug and eroticism. At one time one of our investigators attended a very intimate social gathering in an apartment in Harlem, having succeeded in securing the position of doorman for the occasion. There was a great deal of drinking, and the dancing was of the most modern, abandoned, "jitter-bug" type. This form of dancing is highly suggestive and appears to be associated with erotic activity. The investigator made careful observation of those who were dancing, and found that there was no difference between the ones who were and the ones who were not smoking "reefers." Similar impressions were received after careful observations in public dance-halls, places where they knew that some persons were under the influence of marihuana.

Visits to brothels which occasionally also served as "tea-pads" revealed that the use of marihuana was not linked to sexuality. These observations allow us to come to the conclusion that in the main marihuana was not used for direct sexual stimulation.

Crime

One of the most important causes of the widespread publicity which marihuana smoking has received is the belief that this practice is directly responsible for the commission of crimes.

During our investigation many law enforcement officers, representing various federal, state and local police bureaus were interviewed and asked for a confidential expression of opinion on the general question of crime and marihuana. In most instances they unhesitatingly stated that there is no proof that major crimes are associated with the practice of smoking marihuana. They did state that many marihuana smokers are guilty of petty crimes, but that the criminal career usually existed prior to the time the individual smoked his first marihuana cigarette. These officers further stated that a criminal generally termed as a "real" or "professional" criminal will not associate with marihuana smokers. He considers such a person inferior and unreliable and will not allow him to participate in the commission of a major crime.

In the period beginning October 1939 and ending November 1940, the Police Department made 167 arrests for the possession and use of marihuana. Classified according to race they were: white, 33 men, 4 women; Latin-American, 26 men, 2 women; Negro, 83 men, 6 women; Latin-American (colored) 9 men, 1 woman; British East Indies 1; Filipino 1; Chinese 1.

Classified according to age, 12 per cent were between the ages of 16 and 20, 58 per cent between the ages of 21 and 30, 24 per cent between the ages of 31 and 40, and 6 per cent between the ages of 41 and 50.

During the period under discussion, the Police Department confiscated approximately 3,000 pounds of marihuana.

The sale and use of marihuana is a problem engaging the vigilance of the New York Police Department. However, the number of officers available for such duty is limited. Officers specifically assigned to the Narcotics Division of the Police Department are acquainted with the problem, but the majority of the officers are fundamentally without authoritative knowledge regarding this subject.

The relation between marihuana smoking and the commission of crimes of violence in the city of New York is described by Dr. Walter Bromberg, psychiatrist-in-charge of the Psychiatric Clinic of the Court of General Sessions, in an article published in the *Journal of the American Medical Association:*

"In the south of this country (New Orleans) the incidence of marihuana addicts among major criminals is admittedly high. Sporadic reports from elsewhere in the country of murders and assaults due to marihuana appear in the press frequently. It is difficult to evaluate these statements, because of their uncritical nature. The bulletin prepared by the Foreign Policy Association lists ten cases 'culled at random from the files of the U. S. Bureau of Narcotics' of murder and atrocious assault in which marihuana was directly responsible for the crime. Among the ten patients, the second, J. O., was described as having confessed how he murdered a friend and put his body in a trunk while under the influence of marihuana.

"J. O. was examined in this clinic; although he was a psychopathic liar and possibly homosexual, there was no indication in the examination or history of the use of any drug. The investigation by the probation department failed to indicate use of the drug marihuana. The deceased, however, was addicted to heroin.

"Our observations with respect to marihuana and crime were made in the Court of General Sessions over a period of five and a half years. The material in that court is limited as to residence to New York County, although it must be remembered that the offenders come from many sections of the country and are of many racial types. This is important, because the British investigators have noted in India that cannabis does not bring out the motor excitement or hysterical symptoms in Anglo-Saxon users that occur in natives. There are several other difficulties in collecting reliable material, one being the complete dependence on the history and statements of the prisoners without an opportunity for objective tests or other corroborative check, as in the case of other drugs, e.g., heroin or morphine. During routine interviews of some 17,000 offenders in six and a half years, several hundred have been found who had direct experience with marihuana. Their testimony checks with experimental results and clinical experiences with regard to the symptoms of intoxication, the absence of true addiction and the negative connection with major crime. Especially is this noteworthy among sexual offenders and in cases of assault or murder. The extravagant claims of defense attorneys and the press that crime is caused by addiction to marihuana demands careful scrutiny, at least in this jurisdiction. . . .

"Most of the narcotic cases in New York County are heard in the Court of Special Sessions, where misdemeanants are handled and where indictments on charges of the possession of drugs for use are returned. In the Court of Special Sessions in the same six year period, of approximately 75,000 indictments for all crimes, 6,000 resulted in convictions for the possession and use of drugs. Since neither the law, the district attorney nor the police department makes any distinction between the several kinds of narcotics in arraignments or indictments, there were no figures from which to estimate the number of users of marihuana as distinguished from the number of users of other drugs. A system of sampling the 6,000 cases was therefore adopted in order to furnish an approximate estimate of the total number of marihuana users who came into conflict with the law.

"In this sampling the records of 1,500 offenders, or 25 per cent of the 6,000, were examined. Of these, 135 were charged in connection with marihuana. From this fact it was estimated that about 540 offenders, or 9 per cent of all drug offenders coming to the Court of Special Sessions in six years, were users of marihuana. In analyzing this sample of 135 cases, it was found that ninety-three offenders had no previous record, the previous charge or charges of eight concerned only drugs, five had records including drug charges and twenty-nine had records not including drug charges. Among those with longer records, that is, from four to seven previous arrests, none showed progression from the use of drugs to other crimes.

"As measured by the succession of arrests and convictions in the Court of General Sessions (the only method of estimation) it can be said that drugs generally do not initiate criminal careers. Similarly, in the Court of Special Sessions, only 8 per cent of the offenders had previous charges of using drugs and 3.7 per cent had previous charges of drugs and other petty crimes. In the vast majority of cases in this group of 135, then, the earlier use of marihuana apparently did not predispose to crime, even that of using other drugs. Whether the first offenders charged with the use of marihuana go on to major crime is a matter of speculation. The expectancy of major crimes following the use of cannabis in New York County is small, according to these experiences."[1]

Marihuana and School Children

One of the most serious accusations leveled against marihuana by special feature writers has been that it is widely used by the school children of this nation. These authors have claimed that it has so detrimental an effect on development that it is a major factor in juvenile delinquency. This phase of the marihuana problem was deemed serious enough to merit primary consideration in our study of the marihuana problem in New York City—specifically in the Borough of Manhattan. We decided to attack this aspect of the problem along the following lines:

1. To observe schools in order to see if pupils bought marihuana cigarettes from any peddlers operating in the neighborhood.
2. To investigate thoroughly complaints made by parents to school and police authorities relative to marihuana and its use by school children.
3. To interview principals, assistant principals and teachers of many of the schools in New York City with reference to our project.
4. To gather relevant statistics from various city bureaus and private agencies.

Unknown to the school authorities, our investigators had under surveillance many of the schools in the Borough of Manhattan. They would observe a particular school for a number of consecutive days, watch loiterers and suspicious characters in the locality, and, under certain circumstances, follow some of the children. This procedure was repeated at varying intervals in different localities. From time to time the investigators would return to some of the schools which they previously had kept under surveillance. Attention was naturally concentrated upon those schools from which

(1) Bromberg, W. Marihuana: a psychiatric study. *J. A. M. A. 113:* 4, 1939.

emanated the most numerous complaints and which were located in suspected neighborhoods. We must admit that it would have been possible for such sales to have taken place during the time that our investigators were not on duty, but we came to the conclusion that there was no organized traffic on the part of peddlers in selling marihuana cigarettes to the children of the schools we observed.

Certain of the school authorities deserve special commendation for their alertness in singling out suspicious characters loitering in the vicinity of their schools. While investigating one of the suspected schools, our investigators who were loitering in the neighborhood were suspected and treated as "suspicious characters" by the school authorities.

During the period of this survey the Police Department, while engaged in an entirely separate criminal investigation, received a lead indicating the sale of marihuana to children in a certain high school. As a result, one pupil was arrested and convicted for selling cigarettes to his classmates.

In the Harlem district we discovered a few places where school children gathered during and after school hours for the purpose of indulging in smoking ordinary cigarettes, drinking alcoholic beverages and engaging in homo- and hetero-sexual activities. One of our investigators, having gained entrance to such a place, ostentatiously displayed marihuana cigarettes which he had with him. The madam of the place promptly cautioned him against using the "weed" and insisted that at no time did she permit any person to smoke it on her premises.

A surprising number of school children smoking ordinary cigarettes were noted. A checkup revealed that these cigarettes were being illicitly sold by men on the street and in candy stores in the "loose" form. It is possible that this trade in ordinary cigarettes is occasionally misinterpreted as trade in "reefers."

Interviews with school authorities were very significant, and it is of value to summarize briefly some of the statements actually made by them. The locations of the schools and the names of the persons quoted are in our official files.

1) High School. Predominantly white. The principal stated, "The school has never had any connection with marihuana, not even a rumor."

2) High School. Predominantly white. The principal at first

appeared to be evasive, and did not readily volunteer information, but after repeatedly being pressed with the question stated that the school "had not had any difficulty with the subject of marihuana."

3) High School. Predominantly white. The principal emphatically stated, "I have had no trouble with marihuana in my school."

4) A vocational school in the Borough of Queens. Mixed. "I have never heard the slightest thing about marihuana in connection with this school."

5) High School. Queens. Mixed. "We have never had the slightest connection with marihuana in any way."

6) Junior High School. Harlem. Predominantly Negro and Latin-American. The principal stated that there had been a few marihuana cases among the boys about eighteen months ago. His assistant volunteered the information that there had been some boys in the school who had "reefers" in their possession. On other occasions some of the boys appeared to be intoxicated and when examined confessed to having smoked "reefers." He further stated, "It was difficult to be sure if sleepy, perspiring, pallid-looking boys were feeling the effects of marihuana or were just recovering from too much 'partying' or drinking." He volunteered the opinion that since marihuana was an acute problem among the adult population in that particular district, it could be assumed that marihuana could occasionally become a problem in the school.

7) Junior High School. White and Latin-American. On the fringe of Harlem. Principal and assistant principal stated that they have never had the slightest difficulty arising from marihuana.

8) Junior High School. White and Negro. Bordering on Harlem. The principal, because of his short tenure of office, was unable to express his opinion on the subject. The chief clerk stated that marihuana had never been a problem in the school. She was certain, however, that it was sold in the neighborhood.

9) Junior High School. White, with a high percentage of Negro and Latin-American. The principal stated, "As yet we have had no contact with marihuana although, considering the neighborhood, it would not be unlikely."

10) Junior High School. Latin-American, Negro and some white. The principal stated, "We have had no trouble with marihuana." He was of the opinion that because of the locality it would be possible for some older boys to smoke it without anybody being

cognizant of it. He added that he would let us know if any boys were detected smoking. During the period of the survey no such report was made.

11) Junior High School. Latin-American predominating. The principal stated that she had not had any trouble with marihuana.

12) Junior High School. White predominating. The principal stated, "I have had no contact with it." However, due to the location of the school, which was near Harlem, she stated she would notify the Juvenile Aid Bureau if such a problem arose. During the period of the survey no such report was received.

13) Junior High School. White. The principal stated that no information concerning the use of any narcotics had ever come to his attention and was equally insistent that teachers would have reported any such information to him.

14) Junior High School. White. The principal stated that she had never found anything to indicate the use of any drug in the school.

15) Junior High School. White and mixed. The principal stated that last year he had suspected that a group of chronic truants were using marihuana but he was unable to obtain any direct evidence.

16) Junior High School. White. The principal and his assistant stated that they had no real evidence of any marihuana problem in the school, and they do not believe that the drug is used to any extent.

17) Junior High School. White. The principal stated that although she had no tangible evidence of marihuana smoking among the students, she has problem groups that gather in premises where she is inclined to think that marihuana could be obtained if they wished to get it. She is certain no marihuana is used in the school itself. We investigated thoroughly the suggestions made by the principal as to premises where marihuana might be sold but we were unable to gather any evidence of its sale.

18) Junior High School. White. The acting principal and a teacher in the school who had been there for a number of years stated that there had never been any evidence of the use of marihuana or any other drugs in the school.

19) Junior High School. White. The health director of this school stated that any evidence concerning the use of narcotics by pupils would have been called to his attention, but none had been.

20) Junior High School. White. The authorities stated that there had been no traces of marihuana smoking.

21) Junior High School. White. The authorities stated that there had never been the slightest suggestion of marihuana smoking in the school.

22) Junior High School. White. The assistant principal stated that he knew of no marihuana problem in the school.

23) Junior High School. White. The principal stated that because of the publicity given to marihuana smoking she had been on the alert to discover indications of its use in her school but had found no evidence of marihuana in the school or of anything that would lead her to believe that any one of her students used marihuana outside of the school.

24) Junior High School. White. The principal stated that nothing pertaining to the use of narcotics had been reported to him in all the years he had been there.

25) High School. Predominantly white. Authorities, including the medical department, stated that no student had ever been reported for being under the influence of marihuana.

26) High School. Predominantly white. The principal stated, "There is no indication of a marihuana problem in the school."

27) Grammar School. The principal stated that anonymous letters had been received from time to time from pupils in the school in reference to marihuana. One letter was actually signed by a pupil of the school, who reported the sale of marihuana in a candy store in the vicinity. The principal withheld the name of the pupil but requested us to investigate the report. We kept this school, the immediate neighborhood, and all candy stores in the vicinity, under strict surveillance, but were unable to gather any evidence which would indicate that the pupils of this school were obtaining marihuana.

28) Junior High School. Negro. Queens. The assistant principal stated that he had never heard anything about marihuana being a problem in his school. We had received a complaint about this school and one of our investigators had an informal chat with one of the teachers of this school who, because of her interest in the school children, appeared to be more conversant than anyone else with general problems at the school. She stated that she was certain marihuana was used by some of the students. She elaborated on

the subject and recalled that a few months prior to the interview she had sent home five students (three Negroes and two Italians) whom she had noticed acting "dopey" in the classroom after the noon recess. She was not positive they were under the influence of marihuana but was fairly certain that they were under the influence of some drug. A student had told her that these boys used "reefers" and, noticing their stupor, she had concluded that they were under the influence of marihuana. Superficial examination showed her that their condition was not due to drinking whisky or any alcoholic beverage.

In this school it was not necessary to notify the principal if a student was sent home. The teacher did so on her own account, arriving at a diagnosis without informing the principal of the condition. There was no doctor or nurse to examine the students.

29) Grammar School. Negro. The principal and the social worker attached to this school stated that some time prior to the interview they had heard that cigarettes were being sold to children in Harlem. We were told of a certain man who was suspected of selling them to the children. The social worker was certain that a year before the interview marihuana cigarettes were sold on a certain street in Harlem to school children, but she had no knowledge as to whether the condition existed at the time of our investigation.

While working on another part of the survey, we interviewed a young Negress, approximately 20 years of age, who was a marihuana smoker. She stated that she and another girl started to smoke marihuana cigarettes while attending this particular school.

30) High School. Mixed, predominantly white. The principal stated that he was positive that there was no marihuana problem in his school.

31) High School. Predominantly white. A student was arrested for selling marihuana cigarettes to other pupils. We kept this school under surveillance after the arrest. Although we heard rumors that the sale of marihuana would start again, we were unable to gather any evidence of this. Our investigators attended the dance of the graduating class of this school at one of the hotels in the city. The dance was well conducted and had a large attendance. There was no evidence of smoking at this affair. The principal was cooperating with the Juvenile Aid Bureau of the Police Department in continuing the investigation of the marihuana problem in his school.

32) High School. White and Negro. Although rumor is widespread that "reefer" smoking is common at this school, thorough investigation did not produce evidence of it at the time of our investigation. We did obtain information, which we consider authoritative, that in 1935 a man was offered the concession to sell marihuana cigarettes to the students of this school. He refused the offer. The principal of this school stated that there had never been any trouble as a result of marihuana smoking and he knew of no actual cases.

33) High School. White, Negro and Latin-American. The director of health education who was conversant with the subject stated that the school had no problem with regard to marihuana smoking on the premises but that a Puerto Rican student who lived in Harlem had informed him that he could obtain marihuana cigarettes in his locality.

34) College. White, some Negroes and Latin-Americans. We did not interview the authorities. Observation of the behavior of and conversation with students did not reveal any marihuana problem.

35) College. White, some Negroes and Latin-Americans. This college is located near one of the famous "tea-pads" of Harlem. Many of the students pass the house regularly. Continued observation did not reveal any student attendance.

36) Junior High School. Negro. Most of the boys of this school were familiar with the subject of marihuana. The pupils of the school are incessant smokers of ordinary cigarettes. We were unable to obtain any information which would indicate that they used "reefers." Some students were observed entering a house in which there was a "tea-pad," but we never found any of the occupants of this "tea-pad" to be pupils of the school. The counselor at the school stated that during the previous term there were suspicions regarding the use of marihuana.

37) Junior High School. Negro. The principal, who is considered qualified to discuss this subject, stated that for the three months prior to the interview there had been no marihuana problem. She ventured the opinion that a few cases do arise in the spring and summer. Observation of this school reveals that practically every day young boys between the ages of 18 and 20 loitered near the gates of the school-yard at the close of the session. Some of

these boys were known to our investigators as "reefer" smokers, and they associated with the girls of the school. Two young girls known by our investigators to be "reefer" smokers stated that they started to smoke marihuana while at that school.

38) High School. White, many Negroes and Latin-Americans. Many students smoked ordinary tobacco cigarettes. Numerous complaints and rumors were associated with this school. The principal stated that in 1934 they had had an acute marihuana problem but that at the present time they did not think it existed. They are constantly on guard, especially at the beginning of a term, because they get many new students from the Harlem district. We are of the opinion that there are definite signs indicating that there is some marihuana smoking in the school.

39) High School. Negro and white. The principal of this school stated that they did not have a marihuana problem. We are certain, however, that this school does to some extent present an acute problem for we have observed a few students smoking "reefers" away from the school. We have reason to believe that some of them smoke it while at school. The girls attending this high school have a very low moral standard.

On the basis of the above statements and findings, we feel justified in concluding that although marihuana smoking may be indulged in by small numbers of students in certain schools of New York City, it is apparently not a widespread or large-scale practice.

In the belief that actual facts concerning the role played by marihuana in the production of juvenile delinquency could best be revealed in the records of the Children's Court of New York City, we interviewed the proper authorities on this subject. On the basis of the Children's Court records for 1939, marihuana is not an important factor in the development of delinquency.

Conclusions

From the foregoing study the following conclusions are drawn:

1. Marihuana is used extensively in the Borough of Manhattan but the problem is not as acute as it is reported to be in other sections of the United States.

2. The introduction of marihuana into this area is recent as compared to other localities.

3. The cost of marihuana is low and therefore within the purchasing power of most persons.

4. The distribution and use of marihuana is centered in Harlem.

5. The majority of marihuana smokers are Negroes and Latin-Americans.

6. The consensus among marihuana smokers is that the use of the drug creates a definite feeling of adequacy.

7. The practice of smoking marihuana does not lead to addiction in the medical sense of the word.

8. The sale and distribution of marihuana is not under the control of any single organized group.

9. The use of marihuana does not lead to morphine or heroin or cocaine addiction and no effort is made to create a market for these narcotics by stimulating the practice of marihuana smoking.

10. Marihuana is not the determining factor in the commission of major crimes.

11. Marihuana smoking is not widespread among school children.

12. Juvenile delinquency is not associated with the practice of smoking marihuana.

13. The publicity concerning the catastrophic effects of marihuana smoking in New York City is unfounded.

THE CLINICAL STUDY

Plan and Scope

Interest in the effects of marihuana on the human subject follows two main lines: first, concerning what may be called pleasurable effects which account for its widespread use; and second, regarding undesirable effects, including those leading to criminal and other antisocial acts.

In his monograph on marihuana, Walton has reviewed at length the literature on hashish experience. He has grouped these descriptions as retrospective accounts by professional writers and physicians who have taken the drug through curiosity or scientific interest, reports by physicians concerning patients who have taken excessive doses, and observations by psychiatrists on subjects under marihuana influence. In all of these instances a dose toxic to the individual had been taken and the effects described correspond to psychotic episodes of greater or less degree.

In the literature there are commonly described two basic types of effect, one of excitation, psychic exaltation, and inner joyousness, with divorcement from the external world; the other a state of anxiety with fear of consequences, such as death or insanity. Either one of these types of reaction may be experienced alone, but usually both are present during the intoxication. They occur in no regular sequence but replace each other in rapid succession. The euphoric and anxiety states are generally accompanied by mental confusion, a rapid flow of dissociated ideas, and a feeling of prolongation of time and spatial distortion. Sexual desires or phantasies may also occur.

The detailed descriptions of the experience vary. Those given by trained writers, such as Ludlow and Bayard Taylor, are vivid and dramatic, embodying sensual, visual, and auditory illusions,— phantasies of overpowering splendor and beauty, on the one hand, and intense suffering and horror on the other. The authors, familiar with stories of hashish effects and gifted with strong imaginative powers undoubtedly were expectant of much that happened. The account given by the eminent Philadelphia physician, H. C. Wood, while following the same general pattern, has much less embellishment. He describes a feeling of well-being and inner joyousness and buoyancy and the performance of antics which he knew to be foolish but was unable to control. He was able to recall no illusions or hallucinations. Later a state of anxiety came on, developing into an overpowering fear of death.

A number of studies by psychiatrists on selected subjects have been reported. An excellent example is that of Kant and Krapf. Each acted as subject for the other and the effects of marihuana are described and analyzed at length. In general, the objective in such studies is the interpretation of the reactions in terms of disturbances in psychological processes and functionings.

The descriptions referred to have been given by persons of a higher social class, well-educated and accustomed by training to act in conformity with conventional social behavior. Although a state of irritability may occur and threats of suicide be made by individuals of this type under toxic doses of marihuana, it is noteworthy that in none of the descriptions is there found an expression of antagonism or antisocial behavior which led to acts of violence or what would be called criminal conduct.

Of more direct interest are the publications of Walter Bromberg, psychiatrist, Bellevue Hospital, Psychiatrist-in-Charge, Psychiatric Clinic, Court of General Sessions of New York County. Marihuana users who are brought before the court or admitted to the hospital come under his observation and he has reported at length on the psychiatric observations of 29 of these who showed psychotic reactions. He describes two types of reactions, one an acute marihuana intoxication with a psychotic syndrome, the other a toxic psychosis. Acute intoxication occurs in any individual if the marihuana is taken in sufficiently large doses. It comes on promptly and passes off some hours later. In marihuana psychosis, the symptoms are much more severe and of longer duration. He describes a number of cases in which the psychotic state continued for a number of days and required hospitalization.

The toxic psychosis seen in marihuana users occurs at any time and is of indefinite duration. Bromberg states that the relationship between cannabis and the onset of a functional psychotic state is not always clear. The personality factor is of undoubted importance and other toxic agents such as alcohol and other drugs as well as endogenous elements may be involved. The symptoms, except for the longer duration, resemble those observed in persons under marihuana intoxication, but often take on the characteristics seen in schizophrenic or manic-depressive psychosis.

A description of 11 cases admitted to Bellevue Hospital is given for illustration. The marihuana was taken in the form of cigarettes. In this group were 5 Negroes, 2 of whom were women, 1 Puerto Rican, and 5 whites, one of whom was a Mexican and another a boy of 16. Except for one of the whites, a homosexual, they were all of a low intellectual and social order. One of the Negroes was arrested for following women in Central Park. The others were admitted at their own request, or were sent in by the police or family. Three of the group had definite sexual stimulation but in none was there an outburst in the form of an attack on women. The Puerto Rican became confused and excited and began chasing people with an ice pick. Shortly after his discharge he was readmitted to the hospital, was diagnosed as definitely psychotic, and was transferred to a State hospital as a schizophrenic. The majority of the group, 8 in fact, had psychopathic personalities and 3 of these were transferred to State institutions for further care. The group as a whole is representative of those who come into the hands of the police because of abnormal conduct and who are the source of the sensational newspaper and magazine stories.

Bromberg's findings concerning the lack of a positive relationship between marihuana and crime are described in the sociological section of this study.

In marihuana literature, the action of the drug is usually described from retrospective observation of the effects on a single individual. Relationship to varying dosage, to the subject's personality and background, to environmental conditions when the drug was taken, is given little if any attention. It is the lack of information concerning these and other factors involved in marihuana reaction, which has given rise to the present confusion regarding its effects.

The clinical study here described was designed to afford information not found in marihuana literature but necessary for any comprehensive view of marihuana action. For obtaining this information there were these requisites: an adequate number of subjects for the study, a clear understanding of the mental and physical make-up of each subject, a uniformity of environmental factors, accurately graded dosage of marihuana, and standardized methods of obtaining and recording marihuana effects. In addition to defining the usual and unusual effects of marihuana, as shown by subjective and objective symptoms and alterations in behavior and in physical reaction, the study was expected to answer questions which must arise in consideration of the problem as a whole. Of special importance are these: do marihuana users show fundamental traits differentiating them from non-users; do users present evidence of psychological or physical damage directly attributable to the drug; what are the pleasurable effects which account for the widespread usage of marihuana; to what extent does it lead to antisocial or dangerous behavior?

The sections covering the clinical study are under the following headings:

A. Medical Aspects
   1. Symptoms and Behavior
   2. Organic and Systemic Functions

B. Psychological Aspects
   1. Psychophysical and Other Functions
   2. Intellectual Functioning
   3. Emotional Reactions and General Personality Structure
   4. Family and Community Ideologies

C. Comparison Between Users and Non-Users from the Standpoint of Mental and Physical Deterioration

D. Addiction and Tolerance

E. Possible Therapeutic Applications

Organization for the Study

The clinical studies were carried out at the Welfare Hospital,* a New York City hospital for chronic diseases on Welfare Island. The quarters assigned to the study consisted of a ward of eight beds for the group to be studied at any one period, an adjoining ward of two beds for the study of individuals of the group, three additional rooms with equipment for special examinations, and a diet kitchen for the preparation of the subjects' meals.

Four female nurses were employed and the subjects in the larger ward were under constant supervision. In addition to routine records, each nurse reported the behavior of the subjects while she was on duty. Guards were assigned from the Department of Correction and the New York City Police Force for the subjects drawn from the Riker's and Hart Island penitentiaries and the House of Detention for Women.

The facilities of the Third Medical Division laboratory were

*Now named the Goldwater Memorial Hospital.

used for general clinical laboratory examinations and for more detailed study of organ functioning. For measurement of psychological reactions, special apparatus was provided. A description of equipment used for each division of the study is given under its proper section.

SUBJECTS SELECTED FOR THE STUDY

For the purpose of establishing a uniform plan of procedure to be followed throughout the study, a test group of 5 individuals who had had no previous experience with marihuana was selected. These were volunteers who were paid for their services. They were of a low socio-economic level, but classified as of better than average intelligence. Only one of the group came within the range of what is considered normal personality. They represented the type of person who would readily take to marihuana were the opportunity offered.

The main group, 72 subjects, was drawn from the inmates of the penitentiaries at Riker's and Hart Islands and the House of Detention for Women, all of which are under the supervision of the Department of Correction of New York City. There were two advantages in selecting subjects from this particular group; first, they could be kept under continuous observation throughout the period desired, and second, they constituted an excellent sample of the class in New York City from which the marihuana user comes. The subjects all volunteered for the study after having its purpose and the part they were to take in it fully explained to them.

Race, Sex, and Age. Of the group, 65 were males and 7 were females; 35 were white, 26 were Negros, and 11 were Puerto Ricans. The ages ranged from 21 to 37 years except for one who was 45 and another who was 43. Of the women, 6 had been opium addicts for a number of years.

Previous Experience with Marihuana. Forty-eight of the group, including 6 of the women, gave a history of marihuana smoking. The extent of the usage was variable; for some it was occasional, while others had indulged in the habit fairly steadily over a period of years. Of the 48 users, those who were sellers of marihuana were probably the most consistent smokers, as in carrying on the traffic they would endeavor to keep a stock on hand. But in any instance, the number of cigarettes smoked during any stated period would vary according to circumstance. Thus one user stated that he smoked from 2 to 6 marihuana cigarettes a day, another from 10 to 15 a day, another 3 or 4 a week, and another 5 or 6 a month. Those who smoked daily are here classified as steady users, those who smoked when opportunity was offered but not daily, as occasional users.

TABLE 1

Previous experience with marihuana of 48 subjects

Years of Use	Number of Steady Users	Number of Occasional Users
1–5	13	4
6–10	16	4
over 10	9	2
Total	38	10

The users had all been deprived of marihuana from the time of their arrest, the shortest period being two weeks, the longest, one year and ten months. They all stated that the habit had often been interrupted voluntarily and the enforced discontinuation of it had caused no discomfort.

Health Record. The subjects were individually selected by Dr. Allentuck as suitable for the study. A physical and neurological examination at the hospital showed no evidence of disease. However, the Wassermann and Kline tests gave positive results for 6 subjects and the Kline test alone was positive for 2 and doubtful for 2. These figures are consistent with those of the population from which the group was selected. Of the 12,000 inmates of the Riker's Island Penitentiary in 1940 and the 8,000 in 1941, 10 per cent reacted positively to serological tests.

Intelligence Record. Sixty subjects (40 users and 20 non-users) to whom the Bellevue Adult Intelligence Test was given had an average I.Q. of 99.3, range 70 to 124. The average I.Q. of the user group was 96.7, range 70 to 124, while that for the non-user group was 104.5, range 93 to 114. When analyzed according to racial distribution, the two groups were even better equated intellectually than the total results indicate. Of the 28 white subjects examined, the average I.Q. of the 13 users was 106.1, range 77 to 124, and that of the 15 non-users was 106.3, range 96 to 114. The 19 Negro users had an average I.Q. of 92.6, range 70 to 112, and the 5 Negro non-users averaged 98.8, range 93 to 101. Although in the colored group the non-users averaged 6.2 points higher than the users, it must be taken into account that the number of Negro non-users tested was small. The average I.Q. of the 8 Puerto Rican users was 91.0, range 72 to 100; that is, they were very similar in mental ability to the Negro users. From the results obtained from the Bellevue Adult Intelligence Test, one may conclude that neither the users nor the non-users were inferior in intelligence to the general population.

Marihuana Used

The marihuana that was used for oral administration was supplied by Dr. H. J. Wollner, Consulting Chemist of the United States Treasury Department. It was in the form of an alcohol fluid concentrate, the alcohol content ranging from 55 to 67.3 per cent and the content of solids from 22.9 to 33.6 Gm. per 100 cc. According to the bioassay made by Dr. S. Loewe of the Department of Pharmacology of the Cornell University Medical School, the strength of the fluid concentrate was found to be from 71 to 90 per cent of that of the U.S.P. fluid extract for cannabis marketed by Parke, Davis & Company. The fluid extract was not miscible with water and had a characteristic, disagreeable taste which made it easily recognized. For these reasons the concentrate was evaporated to a viscid consistency and made into pill form, with glycyrrhiza as the excipient. Each pill was equivalent to 1 cc. of the concentrate. For controls, glycyrrhiza pills without marihuana were used.

Several products prepared by Dr. Roger Adams in his investigation of the chemistry of marihuana were used. A comparison of their action with that of the concentrate will be found below.

In addition to the concentrate, marihuana cigarettes were used. These were obtained from supplies confiscated by the New York City Police. Each contained approximately from .4 to .8 Gm. of marihuana. As the quality of the marihuana varied and the amount of active principles taken in with the smoke was unknown, there was no exactness in dosage. In general, however, it appeared that smoking 2 cigarettes was equivalent to taking 1 pill.

The minimal dose of the concentrate which produced clear-cut effects was 2 cc. During the repeated observations on each member of the group larger doses were given, commonly up to around 8 cc. and in one instance up to 22 cc. For smoking, from one to as many as eleven cigarettes were used.

The Active Principles. Determination of relative potencies of drugs having similar action can be made on human beings to a limited extent only. The comparison is based on easily measurable effects on some organ or system on which the drug has a highly selective action, but the existing state of the system influences greatly the ensuing result. Marihuana effects come mainly from action on the central nervous system. The type and degree of response of this system to stimuli of various origins vary in different individuals and in the same individual at different times. When marihuana is given the pre-existing state cannot be classified but it has influence in determining the response, and the same dose of marihuana does not produce identical effects in different subjects or in one subject at different times. In general, however, when the dose given is definitely effective the responses are of a fairly uniform character.

For this reason the relative potency of the active principles supplied by Dr. Roger Adams could be determined only approximately. The principles used were the natural tetrahydrocannabinol, the synthetic isomer, and the synthetic hexylhydrocannabinol. These all brought on effects similar to those of the marihuana concentrate. The estimate of their relative potency is as follows: 1 cc. of the concentrate, representing the extraction from 1 Gm. of marihuana, had as its equivalent 15 mg. of the natural tetrahydrocannabinol, 60 mg. of the synthetic hexylhydrocannabinol, and 120 mg. of the synthetic tetra compound. In explaining the differences in the estimated potencies, the rates of absorption must be taken into account since the action of marihuana depends on the amount of active principle absorbed and its concentration in the brain at a certain time.

The main conclusion is that the action of the marihuana concentrate is dependent on its tetrahydrocannabinol content and that the synthetic compounds retain the action of the natural principle.

Procedure

The procedure for examining the main group of subjects was adopted in the light of the experience gained from the preliminary study.

The subjects were brought to the hospital in groups of from six to ten, and they stayed there from four to six weeks.

Each subject had his history taken and was given a physical, neurological and psychiatric examination on the day of admission. Since it has been shown that pulse variation is the most constant index of marihuana action, the pulse rate was recorded every half hour during the day with the subjects at rest for five minutes before each reading.

During the following days, through careful observation by the Director, the general make-up of the subject, his personality, the character of his responsiveness, and his behavior in new surroundings were determined both before and while he was under the influence of marihuana. Additional information came through the nurses' reports.

In addition, each subject was given a series of tests before and after the administration of marihuana in order that the changes brought about by the drug might be measured. Included among these tests were psychological tests for mental functioning and emotional reactions, psychomotor tests for both simple and complex psychophysical functions, tests to determine such abilities as musical aptitude and the perception of time and space, and laboratory examinations to test the functioning of the various organs and systems of the body.

Medical Aspects

SYMPTOMS AND BEHAVIOR

Samuel Allentuck, M.D.

In Preliminary Group

The preliminary study of the 5 volunteer subjects had for its purpose the establishment of methods of procedures to be followed for the main group, and the obtaining of a general picture of the physical and mental effects induced by the drug. Having no knowledge of the safe limits of marihuana dosage, the dosage given to this group was restricted to from 1 to 4 cc. of the concentrate, and for smoking from 1 to 3 cigarettes.

When ingested, 1 cc. of marihuana was slightly effective, the multiples of this more so. There was noted in all subjects some increase in pulse rate and in blood pressure, dilated and sluggish pupils, dryness of the mouth and throat, ataxia, and some clumsiness and incoordination of movement. Symptoms distinctly disagreeable were dizziness in 3 subjects, a sense of heaviness of the extremities in 2, nausea in 2 and faintness in 2. Three showed motor restlessness. A state classed as euphoria, characterized by laughter, witticisms, loquaciousness, and lowering of inhibitions occurred in 3 subjects. This was not sustained but alternated with periods during which disagreeable symptoms were dominant. In one of the subjects (V.C.) there was no euphoric state, but a feeling of discomfort and depression throughout. Finally in one of the 5 (A.V.) with 2 cc. there was a state of depression with anxiety and with 4 cc. a psychotic episode with fear of death.

With the exception of the one individual during his psychotic episode, the subjects gave no evidence of abnormal mental content at any stage of the drug action, the only change noted being a delay in focusing attention on questions asked and difficulty in sustaining mental concentration. While there was objection at times to carrying out repetitious tests, there was no definite refusal. There was no sexual stimulation giving rise to overt expression.

With the cigarette smoking, ataxia and changes in the pulse rate, blood pressure and pupils corresponded to those following oral administration. In only one of the subjects, however, was there definite euphoria. The common symptoms were dizziness and drowsiness. Two of the subjects found it difficult to concentrate.

The duration of the effects of marihuana was variable. When it was ingested, the effects usually passed off in from two to four hours, but in one instance persisted for seven hours and in another for fourteen hours. After smoking, the duration of effects was from one to three hours.

In Main Group

The evidence of the effects of marihuana was obtained by the subject's statement of symptoms and sensations, by the nurse's reports and by the examiner's observations and interpretation of changes in the subject's mental state and behavior.

The dosage of the marihuana concentrate ranged from 2 to 22 cc. and in each subject the effects of more than one dose were studied. Dosage ranging from 2 to 5 cc. was used for the largest number of subjects, and that from 14 to 21 cc. on only seven occasions. It is known that marihuana intoxication may bring about a comatose state, but no attempt was made to determine the dosage required for this. The number receiving each of the selected doses is shown in Table 2.

TABLE 2

Dosage of marihuana

Dosage	Number of Subjects	Dosage	Number of Subjects	Dosage	Number of Subjects
2 cc.	37	8 cc.	4	14 cc.	1
3 cc.	6	9 cc.	6	15 cc.	2
4 cc.	20	10 cc.	8	17 cc.	1
5 cc.	16	11 cc.	5	18 cc.	1
6 cc.	8	12 cc.	5	19 cc.	1
7 cc.	7	13 cc.	4	22 cc.	1

While the duration of action and its intensity tended to increase with dosage, this was not always the case and equal doses did not bring about uniform effects in all those receiving them. Thus, 3 cc. produced a striking effect in one individual, much less in another; in still another, 10 cc. produced less effect than 5 cc. Such variations are to be explained by differences in the mental make-up of the subject, and the particular state of his responsiveness at the time when marihuana is taken.

The number of cigarettes smoked ranged from one to eleven. The smoking of a single cigarette took about ten minutes and up to eight could be smoked in an hour. In smoking, increasing the number of cigarettes usually increased the sensation described as "high," but here also there was no uniformity in individuals or groups.

When marihuana was ingested, in dosages from 2 cc. up, its actions became evident in from one half to one hour. The maximum effects were seen in from two to three hours. These subsided gradually, but the time of disappearance was variable, usually three to five hours, in some instances twelve hours or more.

When marihuana cigarettes were used the effects appeared almost immediately. After one cigarette, these had usually disappeared in an hour. After several cigarettes had been smoked the effects increased progressively in intensity and reached a maximum in about an hour. In most instances they disappeared in from three to four hours.

The Concentrate

Behavior Symptoms. The effects on the general behavior of the subjects taking the concentrate were variable. If left undisturbed some remained quietly sitting or lying, showing little interest in their surroundings. Others were restless and talkative. Under the heading "Euphoria" there are listed those marihuana effects which give rise to pleasurable sensations or experiences. These are a sense of well-being and contentment, cheerfulness and gaiety, talkativeness, bursts of singing and dancing, daydreaming, a pleasant drowsiness, joking, and performing amusing antics. The drowsiness, daydreaming and unawareness of surroundings were present when the subject was left alone. Other euphoric expressions required an audience and there was much contagiousness of laughing and joking where several of the subjects under marihuana were congregated. The occurrence of a euphoric state, in one or another form, was noted in most of the subjects. But except for those who were allowed to pass the time undisturbed, the pleasurable effects were interrupted from time to time by disagreeable sensations.

Quite commonly seen, as with the preliminary group, was a difficulty in focusing and sustaining mental concentration. Thus, there would occur a delay in the subject's answers to questions and at times some confusion as to their meaning. There was, however, except in a few isolated instances, no abnormal mental content evident and the responses brought out by the examiner were not different from those in the pre-marihuana state.

Altered mental behavior which would give rise to more concern was seen in a relatively small number of subjects. In some this took the form of irritation at questioning, refusal to comply with simple requests and antagonism to certain of the examiners. There was, however, only verbal and no active opposition in any of these behaviors, caused by the subject's desire to be left undisturbed and his disinclination to carry out certain tests which in his pre-marihuana period he had considered tiresome and meaningless. With this came antipathy to those conducting the tests.

The occurrence of the disagreeable physical symptoms accompanying marihuana action would naturally lead to a feeling of disquietude and some alarm as to significance and consequences. This, however, was a prominent feature in relatively few instances. A pronounced state of anxiety reaching a panic stage, associated usually with fear of death or of insanity, was observed only in those subjects experiencing psychotic episodes and here the anxiety state led to pleas for escape and not to acts of aggression. Even in the psychotic states there were no uncontrollable outbursts of rage or acts of violence.

Some evidence of eroticism was reported in about 10 per cent of the 150 instances in which marihuana was administered to the group. The presence of nurses, attendants and other women associated with the study gave opportunity for frank expression of sexual stimulation, had this been marked. There was no such expression even during the psychotic episodes.

In some isolated instances there was evidence of marked lowering of inhibitions such as loud discharge of flatus, urinating on the floor instead of in the vessels supplied and in one instance frank exhibitionism. In the last instance the subject, who was not a regular marihuana user, had been arrested on three occasions for indecent exposure.

The frequency with which significant changes in behavior occurred is indicated in Table 3.

TABLE 3

Effects of varying doses of marihuana on behavior of users and non-users

	2–5 cc.		6–10 cc.		11–22 cc.	
	Per cent affected		Per cent affected		Per cent affected	
Symptoms	Users (41 trials)	Non-users (43 trials)	Users (25 trials)	Non-users (12 trials)	Users (17 trials)	Non-users (3 trials)
Euphoria	92		92		100	
Excitement	19	32	8	41	24	33
Antagonism	7	11	0	16	6	0
Anxiety	7	27	4	41	6	33
Eroticism	4	11	4	16	12	0

As used in Table 3, anxiety means the subject's expressed worry concerning what might happen to him. Excitement, shown by physical restlessness, muscular twitchings and jerky movements, and loud talking, and some degree of antagonism are known to be expressions of an "alarm" or "fear" state.

It is seen from this table that, except for euphoria, the effect of marihuana was definitely more pronounced on the non-users. This might be taken as evidence of a persisting tolerance to the drug in the user group, but, on the other hand, it may have as its basis a feeling of greater apprehension in the non-users. Such a feeling would undoubtedly arise among those who have had no previous experience with marihuana and are in a state of uncertainty as to its possible harmful effects.

Physical Symptoms. Of the subjective symptoms, a feeling described as lightness, heaviness, or pressure in the head, often with dizziness, was one of the earliest and occurred in practically all subjects, irrespective of dose. Dryness of the mouth and throat were reported by over half of the subjects as was also a floating sensation. Unsteadiness in movement and a feeling of heaviness in the extremities were commonly experienced as was a feeling of hunger and a desire for sweets especially. Less commonly noted were nausea, vomiting, sensations of warmth of the head or body, burning of the eyes and blurring of vision, tightness of the chest, cardiac palpitation, ringing or pressure in the ears and an urge to urinate or defecate.

From observation by the examiner, tremor and ataxia were present in varying degrees in practically all instances and in all dosages used, as were also dilatation of the pupils and sluggish response to light. These effects were often present on the day following marihuana administration.

The frequency of the more common subjective symptoms and their relation to dosage is shown in Table 4. The figures are taken from the subjects' reports.

There is a tendency for the symptoms to be more frequent in the non-users than in the users but the differences are variable and in general not striking.

TABLE 4

Physical symptoms produced in users and non-users by varying doses of marihuana

	2-5 cc.		6-10 cc.		11-22 cc.	
	Per cent affected		Per cent affected		Per cent affected	
Symptoms	Users (41 trials)	Non-users (43 trials)	Users (25 trials)	Non-users (12 trials)	Users (17 trials)	Non-users (3 trials)
Lightness in head, dizziness	83	97	80	85	100	100
Dryness of throat	69	72	48	67	76	100
Heaviness of extremities	46	51	32	41	41	67
Unsteadiness	41	39	20	33	41	33
Hunger, thirst	44	35	48	41	70	33
High floating sensation	60	63	72	66	64	33

THE CIGARETTE

Smoking. When marihuana is smoked, there is, as has been stated, no such accuracy in dosage as is the case when it is ingested. The marihuana user acquires a technique or art in smoking "reefers." This involves special preparation of the cigarette and regulation of the frequency and depth of inhalations. In a group of smokers, a cigarette circulates from one to another, each in turn taking one or more puffs. The performance is a slow and deliberate one and the cigarette, held in a forked match stick, is smoked to its end.

When the smoke comes in contact with the respiratory mucous membrane, the absorption of the active principle is rapid and the effects are recognized promptly by the subject. He soon learns to distinguish the amount of smoking which will give pleasant effects from the amount which will give unpleasant ones and so regulates his dosages. Providing there are no disturbing factors, as is the case in gatherings of small friendly groups or parties in "tea-pads," the regulated smoking produces a euphoric state, which accounts for continued indulgence.

The effect from smoking marihuana cigarettes was studied in 32 subjects. Of these, 20 were classed as users, that is, prior to their arrest they had had more or less extensive experience in smoking. In the study the smoking was repeated by each subject several times, the number of cigarettes smoked within an hour ranging from one to eight.

In all of the user group the smoking produced a euphoric state with its feeling of well-being, contentment, sociability, mental and physical relaxation, which usually ended in a feeling of drowsiness. Talkativeness and laughing and the sensation of floating in the air were common occurrences. These effects were of short duration, from one to three or four hours after the smoking was concluded. In none of these subjects was there an expression of antagonism or antisocial behavior.

In the non-user group the effects were similar except that in one subject a state of mental confusion occurred and in another the main effect was a feeling of dizziness, unsteadiness and muscular weakness. Finally one subject showed effects entirely different from the others. He smoked one cigarette and became restless, agitated, dizzy, fearful of his surroundings, afraid of death. He had three short attacks of unconsciousness. At one period he had visions of angels, and for a few minutes a euphoric state. The entire episode lasted a little over an hour after which he went to sleep. This subject had a similar psychotic episode after taking 120 mg. of tetrahydrocannabinol. On seven other occasions he had been given the marihuana concentrate or tetrahydrocannabinol with no unusual effects.

Of the physical symptoms occurring with smoking, dryness of the mouth and throat, dizziness and a sensation of hunger were the most common. None of these or other symptoms seemed to lessen materially the pleasurable effects.

The effect of smoking on the 7 females, 6 of whom were classed as users, corresponded to that on the male group. All showed euphoric effects. One of the subjects was nauseated and another was restless, irritable and contrary. These effects were observed in both of the subjects when marihuana was taken by stomach. One of the users, euphoric after smoking 6 and 10 cigarettes, had a psychotic episode after 8 cc. of marihuana concentrate.

*Tea-Pad Parties.** In addition to the quantitative data regularly obtained from the subject during the course of the testing program, the examiner had opportunity to make diverse observations of the subject's global reactions which threw interesting light on the general effect of the drug on the individual's personality.

When the subject became "high," his inclination was to laugh, talk, sing, listen to music, or sleep, but the requirement that he solve problems, answer questions, or remember drawings created an artificial situation, tending to bring him "down" and spoil his pleasure. In order, therefore, that the influence of the drug might be observed in less formal circumstances and in a set-up more nearly like the customary "tea-pad," two groups of men were given "parties" on the last night of their hospital sojourn. The men were consulted beforehand, and the stage was set according to their desires. They requested that nothing be done until it was really dark outside. They brought the radio into the room where the smoking took place and turned it to soft dance music. Only one shaded light burned, leaving the greater part of the room shadowy. The suggestion was made that easy chairs or floor cushions be procured but the party progressed without these.

The men were allowed as many cigarettes as they wanted. When the "reefers" were passed out they crowded around with their hands outstretched like little children begging for candy. The number of cigarettes the men smoked varied, the range being from two to twelve or thirteen. There were both users and non-users in these two groups. The users of course were highly elated at the prospect of getting much free "tea," and some of the non-users also smoked with genuine enjoyment.

In the beginning the men broke up into little groups of twos and threes to do their smoking, or in some instances went off by themselves. Smoke soon filled the atmosphere and added to the general shadowy effect. After the initial smoking there was some moving about; some men laughed and joked, some became argumentative, while some just stared out of the window. The arguments never seemed to get anywhere, although they often dealt with important problems, and the illogical reasoning used was never recognized or refuted by the person to whom it was addressed. Gradually, as

* This section on "Tea-Pad Parties" was prepared by Mrs. Halpern.

though attracted by some force, all restlessness and activity ceased, and the men sat in a circle about the radio. Occasionally they whispered to one another, laughed a little, or swayed to the music, but in general they relaxed quietly in their chairs. A feeling of contentment seemed to pervade, and when one man suddenly got a "laughing jag" they were annoyed at the interruption.

In general, they gave the impression of adolescent boys doing something which was forbidden and thereby adding spice to the indulgence. Many of the adolescent personality patterns as they appear in group activities were clearly observable here. There was the eternal "wisecracker," the domineering "important" individual who tried to tell everyone what to do, the silly, giggling adolescent and the shy, withdrawn introvert. One forgot that these were actually adults with all the usual adult responsibilities. One could not help drawing the conclusion that they too had forgotten this for the time being.

Although urged to smoke more, no subject could be persuaded to take more than he knew or felt he could handle. After about an hour and a half of smoking, the men were given coffee and bread and jam, and the party broke up. They all went to bed and reported the next day that they had slept very well.

Another attempt at evaluating the effect of marihuana in less formal situations was made in the following manner. The examiner, one of the police officers and the subjects listened to Jack Benny on the Jello Program at 7 o'clock Sunday evening. The police officer noted the number of times the audience laughed, and the length of time the laughter lasted. The examiner checked these items for the subjects. The first time this was done without marihuana; the following week the subjects were given several "reefers" about fifteen minutes before the radio program started. The results were as follows: Without drug, the subjects laughed 42 times as against 72 laughs in the radio audience. The total time for all laughs was 63 seconds as compared with 139 seconds for the radio audience. With cigarettes the subjects laughed 43 times as compared with 47 laughs in the audience, the total laugh time being 129 seconds as compared with 173 seconds of laughter in the audience. Without drug, the subjects laughed, roughly speaking, only half as often and as long as the audience; while under the drug they laughed almost as often and the laugh time was about 75 per cent that of the audience.

It is obvious that under marihuana the subject laughs more readily and for longer time intervals. This is probably due both to the fact that things seem funnier to him and because when under the influence of the drug he is less inhibited.

Differences Between Concentrate and Cigarette

When marihuana was ingested, it was in the form of the concentrate, containing all the active principles which are soluble in the menstruum used. The relative proportions of the principles present are unknown, and the effects can be assumed to give a composite picture of different actions, the dominating one being that of tetrahydrocannabinol. There is no information available concerning the principles present in marihuana smoke, and it is possible that some of those found in the concentrate have been destroyed by the heat of combustion. The effects from smoking correspond to those induced by tetrahydrocannabinol taken by stomach, so it may be assumed that this principle is present in the smoke. The rapidity with which effects occur after smoking demonstrates the quick absorption of the cannabinol from the respiratory tract and the short duration of these effects indicates its prompt excretion or detoxification. When the concentrate is taken, the absorption from the intestinal tract is slower and more prolonged. For these reasons it is not possible to make a precise comparison between the effects of the two forms of administration.

In general the subject's consciousness of unpleasant symptoms is more marked when the concentrate is taken and this may interrupt or obscure the pleasant effects. The long duration of action and the inability of the subject to stop it, serve to accentuate the physical symptoms and to cause apprehension concerning what may happen. The result of all this readily accounts for the irritability, negativism and antagonism occurring. The lessening of inhibitions is not peculiar to marihuana, for in a few subjects who were given alcohol in intoxicating doses the behavior corresponded to that induced by marihuana.

After smoking the main effect was of a euphoric type. Some dizziness and dryness of the mouth were generally present, but were not pronounced enough to distract from the pleasant sensations. The condition described as "high" came on promptly and increased with the number of cigarettes smoked, but it was not alarming or definitely disagreeable, and did not give rise to antisocial behavior. On the contrary it prompted sociability. The marihuana was under the subject's control, and once the euphoric state was present, which might come from only one cigarette, he had no inclination to increase it by more smoking. When a considerable number of cigarettes were smoked, the effect was usually one of drowsiness and fatigue.

The description of the "tea-pad parties" brings out clearly the convivial effect on the groups and the absence of any rough or antagonistic behavior.

Psychotic Episodes

What has been referred to as psychotic episodes occurred in 9 subjects, 7 men and 2 women. A description of the happenings in each instance is given.*

A.V. Male. Non-user. Given 4 cc. of marihuana concentrate. About three hours later he became restless, tremulous, agitated, fearful of harmful effects, suspicious of examiners. For short periods he was euphoric. At one time he had visual hallucinations of figures making gestures suggesting harm. He talked continuously, mainly expressing fear. His answers to questions were delayed but intelligent.

W.P. Male. Occasional user. Given 3 cc., repeated two hours later. At first there was a euphoric state; later he became resistant and negativistic. He showed antagonism to the examiner, demanding to be left alone. He vomited twice. Throughout he was highly excited and talked to himself. The effects in general resembled those seen in a maniacal state. He returned to his normal state in about three hours after the second dose.

F.D. Male. Occasional user. Given 4 cc. Five hours later he became confused, disoriented and slow in answering questions. There were periods of elation and depression with laughter and weeping. The effects passed off in six hours.

R.W. Male. Non-user. Given 5 cc. Three hours later he became disoriented with continued talkativeness and rapid shifting of thought. He had fits of laughter and weeping, grandiose ideas, some paranoid trends. He answered questions clearly but without perseveration. He returned to normal after six hours.

I.N. Female. Occasional user. Also heroin addict for many years. Given 8 cc. Three hours later she became confused and anxious with periods of laughing and weeping. There were several short episodes resembling hysterical attacks with dyspnea, pallor and rapid pulse during which she felt that she was dying and screamed for the doctor and for a priest. Throughout, her response to questioning was intelligent but delayed. There was a return to her normal state in three hours.

E.C. Male. Non-user. Given 6 cc. Two hours later he developed a marked state of anxiety accompanied by a sensation of difficulty in breathing.

* Throughout this section fictitious initials are used to avoid any disclosure of the subjects' identities.

This began during a basal metabolism test. In the Sanborn equipment used there is a nose clip occluding nasal breathing and a rubber mouthpiece through which the air is inspired and expired. During the test the subject became confused, panicky and disoriented as to time. The anxiety over breathing continued for four hours but could be interrupted by distraction. He was then given 4 cc. more. The breathing difficulty lasted five hours more.

The condition here had features seen in claustrophobia. Before the episode the subject had taken marihuana on five occasions in 2, 4, 5, 5, and 2 cc. dosage, without any symptoms of respiratory distress. However, after the episode he took marihuana on three occasions in 2, 5, and 6 cc. dosage and each time the respiratory symptoms occurred. A certain degree of nervousness was present but there was no mental confusion. The subject realized that there was no physical obstruction to his breathing and had learned that by concentrating his thought on other lines he could keep his respiratory difficulties in abeyance and would not suffer from real anxiety. Smoking up to as many as thirteen marihuana cigarettes did not bring about the respiratory effect. It appeared then that the respiratory symptoms were precipitated by the wearing of the apparatus while under the influence of marihuana, and through suggestibility there resulted a conditioning to the marihuana concentrate which was given subsequently.

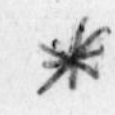

The description of these six psychotic episodes fits in with many others found in marihuana literature. They are examples of acute marihuana intoxication in susceptible individuals which comes on shortly after the drug has been taken and persists for several hours. The main features of the poisoning are the restlessness and mental excitement of a delirious nature with intermittent periods of euphoria and an overhanging state of anxiety and dread.

Three other subjects presented the features of marihuana psychosis.

R.H. Male. White. Age 23. Non-user. In prison for the offense of living on prostitution. The family history was bad. His father never supported his wife or family and there was continual discord at home. When the subject was 9 years old the father deserted the family. Three brothers received court sentences, one for stealing a taxi, one for rape, and one for striking a teacher. R.H. was a problem child at school and on account of truancy and waywardness he was sent to the Flushing Parental School. He ran away from this school several times and was transferred to the House of Refuge on Randall's Island. At the age of 16 he was discharged. Since that time he had had two jobs, one for three months in a factory, the other for four and one-half months in the W.P.A. When he was 16 he was run over by a truck and was unconscious for a time. After his return to the Riker's Island Penitentiary from Welfare Hospital further questioning concerning his past revealed that he was subject to "fits" occurring once or twice every two months. During the attacks his body became rigid and his mouth felt stiff.

The subject was admitted to Welfare Hospital for the marihuana study on February 20th. After the usual program of examinations he was given 2 cc. of the concentrate on February 27th and February 28th. These doses brought on the symptoms of dizziness and tremor and heaviness of the head and the state called "high" which is characterized by periods of laughter and talkativeness. These effects passed off in a few hours and were followed by drowsiness and a sense of fatigue. On March 1st at 1 p.m. he smoked one marihuana cigarette. Immediately afterwards he became agitated and restless and suddenly lost consciousness. He recovered quickly and stated that he had had visions of angels and had heard choirs singing. Later he had a second short period of unconsciousness. During the afternoon he continued to be agitated and restless and had periods of laughing and weeping. After he was given phenobarbital he went to sleep. On the next day his only complaint was that he felt dizzy. Following this episode he was given 4 cc. of marihuana concentrate on March 3rd and 2 cc. on March 10th and 2 cc. of tetrahydrocannabinol on March 5th and 4 cc. on March 8th. The effects corresponded to those seen after the earlier administrations of 2 cc. doses of the concentrate.

On March 11th R.H. was given 5 cc. (75 mg.) of the tetrahydrocannabinol at 11 a.m. and 3 cc. at 2 p.m. No unusual effects were noted during the afternoon and he ate his supper with appetite at 4:30 p.m. At 6 p.m. he became restless, apprehensive and somewhat belligerent. He felt that something had happened to his mother, that everybody was acting queerly and picking on him. He continued to be agitated and fearful, refused medication and slept poorly. This condition persisted and on March 13th he was returned to Riker's Island. After four days there he became quiet and composed. The psychotic state cleared up completely. The resident psychiatrist's report was: Impression 1. Psychosis due to drugs. (Marihuana experimentally administered.) Acute delirium, recovered. 2. Convulsive disorder, idiopathic epilepsy. Petit mal on history.

H.W. Female. White. Age 28. Non-user. Drug peddler, serving three years' indefinite sentence for unlawfully possessing a drug. Her parents died when she was about 10 years old and she was raised in an orphanage. At the age of 19 she entered a training school for nurses, but gave this up after four months and supported herself by prostitution. Her sister and her sister's husband were drug addicts and through them she began taking morphine and heroin, being, according to her account, depressed and dissatisfied at the time. She continued using these drugs up to the time of her arrest, a period of eight years. In 1938 she married a man who was also a drug addict, and engaged in the drug traffic.

On May 7th she was given 2 cc. of marihuana. Aside from a headache and a feeling of muscular weakness and incoordination, the effect was to make the subject feel gay and very good-natured. On May 8th she was given 3 cc. of the concentrate and became somewhat confused and unsteady, irritated and upset at carrying out tests, and greatly worried about the physical symptoms. Five hours after she had taken the drug the effects had largely passed off. Six hours later, however, she became restless and agitated, moving about constantly, and worried about past conduct. This state continued for a few hours. On other occasions the subject was given marihuana in doses of 2, 3, and 4 cc. Twice after the administration of 3 cc. the general effect was of a euphoric type, and after 4 cc. had been given a state of sadness set in on two occasions and one of euphoria on a third. Toward the end of her stay the subject became depressed and moody, constantly dwelling on the belief that she had committed unpardonable sins.

She was returned to the House of Detention on June 2nd, transferred to the Psychiatric Division of Bellevue Hospital on June 9th, and from there was sent to Matteawan State Hospital on July 10th. On admission to the State Hospital she appeared confused, retarded, apprehensive, and depressed. She had a marked feeling of guilt. She began to improve in September and was discharged, cured, in January. Since her return to New York she reports at frequent intervals to the parole officer. She has secured employment in a food shop and is to be promoted to the position of manager of the shop.

The diagnosis made at the State Hospital was: Psychosis, due to drugs and other exogenous poisons (morphine and heroin).

D.P. Male. Colored. Age 23. Occasional user. Sentenced for unlawful possession of drugs. Since graduation from high school at the age of 16 he had had no occupation. His criminal record dated from his graduation. He was arrested in 1934 for disorderly conduct and in the same year sentenced to Elmira Reformatory for five years for second degree assault. He was paroled in 1936, but during the same and the following year was arrested three times for assault or robbery. He was returned to Elmira where he remained until his discharge in 1940. In August 1940 he was arrested for the possession of drugs and sentenced to a three-year indefinite term. He had served eight months of this sentence when he was admitted to Welfare Hospital as a subject for the marihuana study.

During his stay at Welfare Hospital, D.P. was given marihuana in the form of a concentrate and as cigarettes on numerous occasions. His symptoms and behavior corresponded to those usually seen, lasting a few hours with no after-effects. When the time came for his return to Riker's Island he urged that he be allowed to stay at the hospital and assist in the study. Two weeks after his return to the penitentiary he developed a psychosis characteristic of schizophrenia. He was transferred to Matteawan where the diagnosis made was: Psychosis with psychopathic personality.

These three cases are of special interest from the standpoint of the relationship of marihuana to the psychosis. The first subject, R.H., had a definite history of epileptic attacks. After smoking one marihuana cigarette he experienced an acute confusional state which lasted a few hours. In the second episode which lasted six days there was a more prolonged confusional state. Epileptics are subject to
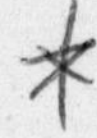
such attacks, epileptic or epileptic equivalents, which may be brought on by any number of upsetting circumstances. In this case marihuana is the only known factor which precipitated the attack.

The second subject, H.W., was a heroin addict of long standing. During her stay in the hospital, in her retrospective reports on her marihuana experiences there were usually included expressions of worry and remorse at her conduct, such as her failure to answer questions or perform tests honestly, informing on the other women in her group, and denials concerning a syphilitic infection she thought she had had. Prior to this incarceration she had had no prison experience. The mental picture developed from the study at the hospital and at Matteawan and the subject's subsequent history represent a fairly typical example of what is termed a prison psychosis.

The third subject, D.P., did not develop his psychosis until two weeks after he had been returned to the Riker's Island Penitentiary. He had shown no unexpected effects from marihuana and had hoped to be allowed to stay on at the hospital instead of going back to prison to complete more than two years of an unexpired sentence. At Matteawan this subject was considered to have an underlying psychopathic personality. His case also may be taken as an example of prison psychosis. With both the second and third subjects, the exact role of marihuana in relation to the psychosis cannot be stated.

Dr. Peter F. Amoroso, Commissioner of Correction of the city of New York, has given us information concerning the prisoners sentenced to the penitentiary at Riker's Island from whom our subjects were drawn. During the year beginning July 1, 1941 and ending June 30, 1942, there were 1,756 inmates in this institution. They had received an indeterminate sentence, that is, from a minimum of a few months to a maximum of three years. Of this group, 175 were subjected to intensive study by the psychiatrist because they were considered possible psychotic cases, 117 were sex offenders, and 200 were miscellaneous cases referred for mental observation, making a total of 492. Twenty-seven of these cases were committed to state institutions for the criminal insane, namely, 25 to Matteawan and 2 to Dannemora.

Commissioner Amoroso, after reviewing these cases, writes as follows: "The prison atmosphere may place a most severe strain on those who are physically or mentally abnormal upon commitment . . . Emotionally unstable persons find themselves during incarceration denied the assertion and enjoyment of the basic human urges and impulses and it is natural to expect, therefore, that prison life may result in various types of explosions, such as psychoses, neuroses, sex perversion, and even physical and moral deterioration.

"I am indeed surprised that we had so little trouble with our volunteers upon completion of their study and sojourn at Welfare Hospital, and the few psychotic episodes that occurred are exactly what we would expect in the whole group without considering the administration and effects of excessive doses of marihuana."

SUMMARY

In the study of the actions of marihuana in respect to subjective and objective symptoms and behavior, the marihuana was given a number of times to each of the subjects in the form of the concentrate taken by stomach. The amount given ranged from 2 to 22 cc., in most cases from 2 to 5 cc. After marihuana was taken, the systemic action became evident in from one-half to one hour and the maximum effects were seen in from two to three hours. They passed off gradually, usually in from three to five hours, although in some instances they did not completely disappear until twelve or more hours.

Of the symptoms occurring, a feeling of lightness in the head with some dizziness, a sensation of floating in the air, dryness of the throat, hunger and thirst, unsteadiness and heaviness in the extremities were the most frequent. Tremor and ataxia, dilation of the pupils and sluggishness in responsiveness to light were observed in all subjects.

From observations on the behavior and responses of the subjects, it was found that a mixture of euphoria and apprehension was generally present. If the subjects were undisturbed there was a state of quiet and drowsiness, and unawareness of surroundings, with some difficulty in focusing and sustaining mental concentration. If they were in company, restlessness, talkativeness, laughter and joking were commonly seen. A feeling of apprehension, based on uncertainty regarding the possible effects of the drug and strengthened by any disagreeable sensations present, alternated with the euphoria. If the apprehension developed into a state of real anxiety, a spirit of antagonism was shown. However any resistance to requests made to the subjects was passive and not physical and there was no aggressive or violent behavior observed. Erotic ideas or sensations when present took no active expression.

Six of the subjects developed toxic episodes characteristic of acute marihuana intoxication. The dosage varied from 4 to 8 cc. of the concentrate, and the episodes lasted from three to six hours, in one instance ten hours. The effects were mixtures of euphoric and anxiety states, laughter, elation, excitement, disorientation and mental confusion.

The doses given were toxic to the individuals in question but not to others taking the same or larger ones. Once the drug had been taken the effects were beyond the subject's control. The actions described took unusual expression because for the particular subject at a particular time the dose was unusually effective. A corresponding toxicity did not occur from cigarettes for here the effects came on promptly and on the appearance of any untoward effects, the smoking was stopped.

In three of the subjects a definite psychotic state occurred, in two shortly after marihuana ingestion, in one after a two-week interval. Of the first two, one was an epileptic and the other had a history of heroin addiction and a prepsychotic personality. The third was considered a case of prison psychosis. The conclusion seems warranted that given the potential personality make-up and the right time and environment, marihuana may bring on a true psychotic state.

ORGANIC AND SYSTEMIC FUNCTIONS

Samuel Allentuck, M.D.

The functions of the body organs and systems were studied in the manner common to hospital practice according to the methods and with the equipment in use at Welfare Hospital. The study was designed to show not only the effects of varying doses of marihuana but also whether subjects who had long been users of the drug gave evidence of organic damage. The tests were made before the drug was administered, during its action, and often in the after period. The heart and circulation, blood composition, kidney, liver and gastro-intestinal function, and basal metabolism received special consideration. The results of the study follow.

The Circulation

Pulse Rate

Coincident with the onset of marihuana symptoms, there usually occurred a rise in pulse rate. The peak was reached in from one and 

one-half to three and one-half hours. The maximum increase was from 30 to 40 beats per minute in most instances but in some it was from 50 to 60 beats. The decline after the peak was at times sharp, at other times gradual. The rise and its extent appeared to be dependent upon the mental state induced by the drug, that is, it was greater in states of euphoria with talkativeness, laughter, and body movement. As these symptoms subsided the pulse rate fell correspondingly.

Blood Pressure

Blood pressure changes were variable. In general, there was a rise in blood pressure coincident with the increase in pulse rate. There was no consistency in this, however. Thus, in one instance, with an increase of 30 beats per minute in pulse rate, the blood pressure rose 20 mm. Hg.; in another, with a rise in pulse rate of 50 beats per minute, the blood pressure remained unchanged. The diastolic pressure in general followed the systolic. There was no consistent relationship between the degree of change and the size of dosage.

Circulation Time

In a number of instances, ether and saccharin were injected into the antecubital vein and the time intervals required for the recognition of ether in the expired air and of the taste of saccharin were measured. The measurements made before and during marihuana action showed no differences and it was concluded that marihuana has no effect on the arm to lung and arm to tongue circulation time.

Electrocardiograms

Electrocardiographic records were made of all subjects before the administration of marihuana and during the drug action. The dose ranged from 1 cc. upwards, going as high as 17 cc. for one subject. In a number of instances a preliminary dose was given in the morning and a second, usually much larger one, later, the record being taken after the second dose. The readings and interpretations were made by Dr. Robert C. Batterman.

In 11 of the subjects abnormal electrocardiograms were noted. A description of these follows:

A.B.	Control	P split in leads 2 and 3.
	Marihuana	same
T.E.	Control	P split in leads 2 and 3. Left axis deviation.
	Marihuana	same throughout
C.H.	Control	T diphasic in leads 1 and 2.
	Marihuana	T diphasic in leads 2, 3 and 4.
J.H.	Control	Normal PR interval .18.
	Marihuana	P split in leads 1, 2 and 3. PR interval .22.
W.J.	Control	Elevated ST segment, lead 1 and 4. P split in leads 1, 2 and 3. T diphasic in 3. P diphasic in lead 4.
	Marihuana	LA deviation. P split in leads 1, 2 and 3. T inverted in lead 3.
J.P.	Control	P split in leads 1, 2 and 3. Diphasic in lead 4. T split in 2, diphasic in 3.
	Marihuana	P split in 2.
J.R.	Control	RA deviation, P split in lead 1.
	Marihuana	RA deviation, P split in leads 1 and 2.
C.S.	Control	Deep Q in lead 3. Inverted T in lead 3. Depressed ST segment lead 2.
	Marihuana	same throughout
L.V.	Control	Ventricular rate 120. RA deviation. P split in leads 1, 2, 3 and 4. PR interval .20.
	Marihuana	Ventricular rate 120. No deviation. P split in leads 1, 2, 3 and 4. PR interval .24.
B.W.	Control	Normal
	Marihuana	Sinus tachycardia. T inverted in leads 3 and 4.
H.W.	Control	T split in leads 1, 2 and 3. P inverted in lead 3. Wassermann positive.
	Marihuana	same throughout

In 9 of the subjects, 7 users and 2 non-users, abnormal electrocardiograms were noted in both the readings taken before and those taken after the administration of marihuana. In 4 of these the tracings resemble the pattern of those seen in patients with rheumatic heart disease, but it is impossible to state what underlying pathological conditions were present in the group as a whole. In 2 users the control records were normal, the marihuana ones abnormal.

In 6 subjects not included in the list given, a sinus tachycardia, and in 2 a sinus bradycardia were seen after the ingestion of marihuana.

In all the remaining subjects no abnormalities were seen before or during marihuana action.

Hematology

Blood morphology and certain chemical constituents of the blood were studied before and during marihuana action on 61 subjects, the dosage ranging from 2 to 21 cc. Before the administration of marihuana the hemoglobin reading was between 80 and 90 per cent in 36 subjects and over 90 per cent in 22; during marihuana action it was from 80 to 90 in 19 subjects and over 90 per cent in 39. Three showed a low hemoglobin percentage before, 65, 70 and 77 per cent, but a rise to 79, 90, and 95 per cent during the drug action.

The blood counts showed the usual individual variations but the average counts for the 61 subjects were: before the administration of the drug, red blood cells 4,800,000 and white blood cells 8,900; during the drug action, 4,900,000 and 9,500 respectively.

The urea nitrogen, calcium and phosphorus blood concentration figures are given in Table 5.

TABLE 5

Blood concentrations of urea nitrogen, calcium and phosphorus (in milligrams per cent)

	Number of Subjects	Before Marihuana		After Marihuana	
		Average	Range	Average	Range
Urea nitrogen	63	12.2	6.9–24.9	12.2	8.5–20.7
Calcium	39	11.2	10.2–13.2	11.2	10.0–12.5
Phosphorus	36	3.9	2.6– 5.5	3.7	2.8– 5.0

From these blood studies it is seen that marihuana in the range of dosage stated produced no appreciable change in hemoglobin or

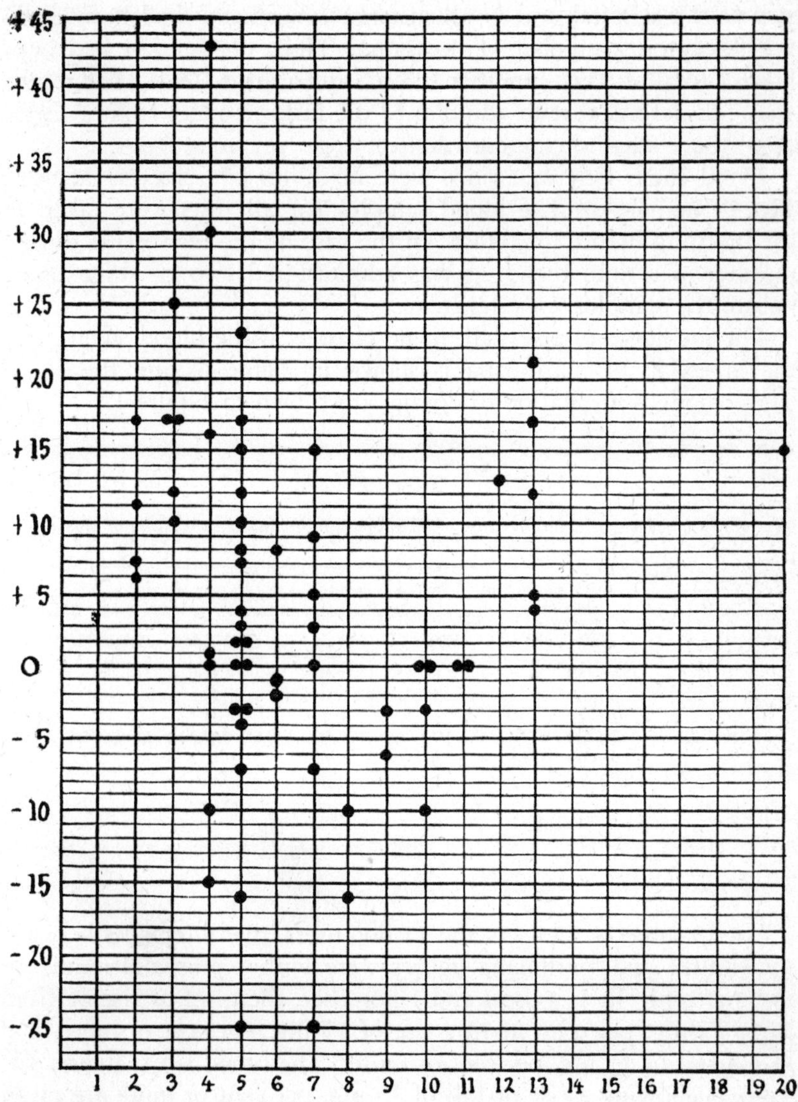

FIGURE 1. Increase or Decrease in Blood Sugar of Sixty-Two Subjects as a Result of Varying Doses of Marihuana.

cell count or in blood urea, calcium, and phosphorus. The blood examinations were made at varying periods during the subjects' stay at the hospital and in all instances marihuana had been given previously on a number of occasions. Thus, one subject had been given a total of 85 cc., another 143 cc., and a third 169 cc. The results show, therefore, that in addition to the lack of effect from a single dose, there was no cumulative effect from previous doses.

Blood sugar determinations were made on 62 subjects, 42 users and 20 non-users. The blood samples for all tests were taken in the morning before breakfast. In the case of the tests made during marihuana action, the drug was administered two or three hours before the samples were taken.

The incidence of rise, fall, or no change in the blood sugar after the ingestion of marihuana is shown in Table 6, and the blood sugar changes in relation to dosage are shown in Figure 1.

TABLE 6

Changes in blood sugar determination of 62 subjects following the ingestion of marihuana

Blood Sugar before Marihuana (in mg. %)	Number of subjects showing		
	Rise	Fall	No change
55–59.....	1	0	0
60–69.....	3	0	0
70–79.....	7	1	0
80–89.....	19	9	5
90–99.....	5	6	2
100–110.....	1	2	1
Total...	36	18	8

For 38 subjects, 27 users and 11 non-users, the differences between the control and marihuana figures were within plus and minus 10 mg. per cent. In 5, 4 users and 1 non-user, there was a rise of from 11 to 14 mg. per cent, in 14 a rise of 15 mg. per cent or more, and in 5 a fall of 15 mg. per cent or more. The blood sugar figures for subjects showing a rise or fall of 15 mg. per cent or more are given in Table 7.

TABLE 7

Blood sugar changes of 15 milligrams per cent or more

15 mg. % or more rise				15 mg. % or more fall			
Dose	Before Marihuana	After Marihuana	Differ-ence	Dose	Before Marihuana	After Marihuana	Differ-ence
Users				*Users*			
A.R. 20 cc.	85	100	15	J.W. 8 cc.	90	74	−16
W.J. 13 cc.	91	108	17	J.H. 5 cc.	98	73	−25
J.N. 13 cc.	91	112	21	J.B. 4 cc.	85	70	−15
W.C. 5 cc.	55	78	23				
B.W. 5 cc.	73	90	17				
J.T. 5 cc.	85	100	15				
W.S. 4 cc.	89	105	16				
W.R. 4 cc.	60	90	30				
Non-users				*Non-users*			
E.F. 7 cc.	90	105	15	A.T. 7 cc.	105	80	−25
L.V. 4 cc.	82	125	43	S.L. 5 cc.	100	84	−16
C.C. 3 cc.	68	85	17				
W.H. 3 cc.	75	92	17				
P.B. 3 cc.	75	100	25				
J.T. 2 cc.	83	100	17				

From these tables it is seen that while there was a trend toward a rise in blood sugar levels during marihuana action, for the majority of the subjects there was no significant change from the control levels. In the instances where a rise or fall of 15 mg. per cent or more occurred, a level of over 100 mg. per cent was noted in only 5 subjects under marihuana; in the 14 others the range kept between 70 and 100 mg. per cent, which may be considered normal limits. Throughout there was no distinction between users and non-users in regard to blood sugar levels.

The Kidney

Routine examinations of twenty-four-hour urine specimens were made on all subjects for periods before and following marihuana administration. In no instance were albumin, sugar, casts, blood cells or other abnormal elements found.

Thirty-six subjects were given 1,000 cc. of water and the urine was collected for three one-hour periods. The procedure was repeated after the administration of marihuana in doses varying from 2 to 13 cc. An analysis of the figures obtained gave no evidence of a diuretic or antidiuretic effect from marihuana.

It was observed that an urge to urinate was a not infrequent occurrence during marihuana action. Since this was not accompanied by any appreciable increase in the amount of urine output, it is probable that it was a psychological reaction.

The phenolsulfonphthalein test for kidney function was carried out on 49 subjects before and during marihuana action. The dose ranged from 4 to 17 cc. The results are shown in Table 8.

TABLE 8

Phenolsulfonphthalein Test. Number of subjects excreting various percentages of injected solution in two hours

Period	Number of Subjects Excreting Under 40%	40-49%	50-59%	Over 60%
Before Marihuana	13	13	15	8
After Marihuana	16	13	13	7

There was a decrease of 2.5 per cent in the total amount excreted by the 49 subjects after the administration of marihuana as compared with the amount excreted under normal conditions. This difference is well within the limits of technical error.

The results of the examinations showed therefore that the administration of marihuana brought about no structural or functional change in the kidney as determined by the techniques employed.

The Liver

No clinical evidence of liver damage was observed in any of the subjects before or after marihuana had been administered. The bromsulfalein test was given to a number of the subjects. The dye was injected in amounts of between 2 and 3 mg. for each kilogram of weight and the blood examined after thirty minutes. In 20 instances where marihuana was given in dosage ranging from 2 to 10 cc. and in 1 instance where 20 cc. was administered, the dye was absent from the blood after the thirty-minute interval.

The Gastro-Intestinal Tract

As has been stated, a characteristic effect of marihuana is a sensation of hunger and an increased appetite. Disagreeable effects which may occur are nausea and vomiting. The frequency with which the symptoms were noted is given in Table 9.

TABLE 9

Gastro-intestinal symptoms

Dose	Number of subjects	Number of trials	Symptoms			
			Hunger	Nausea	Vomiting	Diarrhea
Concentrate						
	Men					
1– 3 cc.	64	184	94	5	2	occurred in 4 of the psychotic episodes
4– 5 cc.	59	186	129	7	2	
6– 8 cc.	46	106	85	6	3	
9–22 cc.	33	71	50	2	1	
	Women					
1– 3 cc.	7	28	17	6	1	
4– 6 cc.	7	35	25	1	0	
7–10 cc.	4	5	3	0	0	
Cigarettes						
	Men					
1–8.	37	54	40	3	1	
	Women					
1–8.	5	7	5	2	1	
Tetrahydrocannabinol (natural and synthetic)						
	Men					
	34	93	61	7	5	
	Women					
	6	18	11	2	2	

As shown in the table, after the ingestion or smoking of marihuana more than half the subjects experienced hunger and increased appetites. A desire for sweets was especially strong, and users believe that the taking of candy or sweetened drinks lessens the "too high" effect which may follow marihuana smoking. The tendency toward a rise in blood sugar after the ingestion of marihuana indicates some need of the tissues for more sugar, but there is no explanation of the mechanisms involved.

While nausea and vomiting might be attributed to irritant effects of marihuana, on the other hand these symptoms occurred after smoking and in one instance after an intramuscular injection of tetrahydrocannabinol. The action here is presumably a central one.

The effects of marihuana on gastric motility and secretion were studied by Dr. Louis Gitzelter. A Miller-Abbott balloon attached to a Levine tube was passed into the stomach through one nostril and a Levine tube alone through the other nostril. The balloon was inflated with air to a pressure of approximately 10 mm. of water and connected with a tambour which registered gastric contractions on a kymograph. The other Levine tube was used to withdraw gastric contents at stated periods.

With the subjects in a fasting state, control records of gastric motility and measurements and analyses of gastric secretion were made throughout a period of an hour or more. The procedure was repeated on subsequent days following the administration of marihuana (6, 8, 6, 15, and 15 cc.) and at a time when the subjects were in a "high" state. A comparison of the two sets of findings gave no evidence that marihuana had any effect on motility or brought about any change in gastric secretion.

Roentgenograms, which were taken of the stomach of one of the subjects after a barium test meal, showed the emptying time of the stomach to be three hours both before and after the administration of marihuana. In another subject there was considerable delay in the emptying time during the marihuana action.

The Brain

Brain Metabolism

The effect of marihuana on the metabolic rate of the brain was investigated by studying the oxygen and carbon dioxide content of the arterial and venous blood drawn from the carotid artery and the internal jugular vein. The blood samples were obtained as simultaneously as possible, collected under mineral oil, and kept under anaerobic conditions until analyzed. Coagulation was prevented by the use of oxalate, and glycosis was inhibited by the addition of fluoride. The blood samples were analyzed for oxygen and carbon dioxide by the method of Van Slyke and Neil.

For analyses made when the subjects were under the influence of marihuana, the blood samples were collected two and a half or three hours after the drug was given, at a time when the subjects were in a state classed as "high."

The results presented in Table 10 show no consistent change in the metabolism of brain tissue as measured by blood oxygen and carbon dioxide concentration in 4 subjects showing clinical evidences of marihuana intoxication. Circumstances prevented an extension of the study.

TABLE 10

Oxygen and carbon dioxide content of arterial and venous blood of four subjects before and after the administration of marihuana

		Oxygen content			Carbon dioxide content		
		Arterial blood (in volume per cent)	Venous blood	Difference	Arterial blood (in volume per cent)	Venous blood	Difference
Before Marihuana	R.S.	19.3	14.3	5.0	48.6	52.0	3.4
	M.G.	19.4	14.9	4.5	46.7	50.8	4.1
	A.B.	20.4	16.3	4.1	45.2	50.8	5.6
	W.S.	19.4	13.7	5.7	45.4	52.9	7.5
After Marihuana	R.S.	19.1	10.7	8.4	46.8	55.0	8.2
	M.G.	20.2	14.9	5.3	44.2	48.5	4.3
	A.B.	20.2	14.9	5.3	43.3	48.4	5.1
	W.S.	18.0	12.9	5.1	47.0	49.0	2.0

ELECTROENCEPHALOGRAMS

Electroencephalographic records of 15 subjects were made by Dr. Hans Strauss. There appeared to be a relationship between the typical euphoric reaction produced by marihuana and an associated increase in the alpha activity seen in the electroencephalogram. However, similar increase of alpha activity was observed in 2 subjects who received no marihuana. It is known that a high degree of alpha activity is suggestive of relaxation or perhaps the shutting off of any disturbing extraneous environmental stimuli and these findings merely suggest that marihuana is conducive to mental relaxation in some individuals.

Basal Metabolism

The basal metabolic rates of 61 subjects were determined before and during marihuana action. The Sanborn apparatus was used and the determinations were made in the morning before breakfast. The marihuana dosage ranged from 2 to as high as 20 cc. In the group of 61 subjects, 45 were classed as users, 16 as non-users. The accompanying table gives the data on 43 subjects whose metabolic rates were within a range of +9 to −13 per cent, both under normal conditions and while under the influence of marihuana. Of these, 19 showed a rise in basal metabolic rate of from 2 to 12 per cent, 23 a fall of from 2 to 13 per cent, and in 1 the rate did not change.

TABLE 11

Metabolic rates (in per cent) within a range of from +9 to −13 per cent

Dose	Without Marihuana	Under Marihuana	Difference	Dose	Without Marihuana	Under Marihuana	Difference
Users				*Users*			
H.W. 10 cc.	− 2	+ 5	+ 7	A.R. 20 cc.	0	− 8	− 8
W.C. 8 cc.	− 6	0	+ 6	E.T. 17 cc.	− 7	−11	− 4
C.J. 8 cc.	+ 4	+ 5	+ 1	J.B. 13 cc.	− 4	−13	− 9
J.H. 8 cc.	−13	+ 4	+17	W.J. 13 cc.	0	− 8	− 8
R.T. 7 cc.	− 7	0	+ 7	R.S. 13 cc.	0	− 4	− 4
L.C. 6 cc.	−12	−10	+ 2	A.B. 11 cc.	− 5	−11	− 6
P.B. 6 cc.	− 5	− 2	+ 3	J.W. 8 cc.	− 3	− 5	− 2
F.W. 6 cc.	−11	− 7	+ 4	O.D. 7 cc.	+ 4	− 6	−10
M.N. 5 cc.	− 9	− 5	+ 4	M.V. 6 cc.	− 5	−10	− 5
S.L. 5 cc.	− 9	+ 2	+11	J.R. 5 cc.	− 7	−10	− 3
A.B. 4 cc.	−12	0	+12	W.B. 5 cc.	− 6	−13	− 7
W.S. 4 cc.	− 5	+ 7	+12	H.W. 5 cc.	− 9	−13	− 4
R.S. 4 cc.	− 9	− 5	+ 4	M.G. 5 cc.	− 2	− 5	− 3
M.B. 2 cc.	− 2	+ 5	+ 7	K.S. 4 cc.	+ 9	− 5	−14
C.D. 2 cc.	−12	0	+12	M.S. 2 cc.	− 2	− 7	− 5
				A.S. 2 cc.	+ 4	− 2	− 6
Non-users				*Non-users*			
D.L. 10 cc.	+ 5	+ 7	+ 2	W.B. 7 cc.	− 6	− 4	− 2
L.V. 6 cc.	− 2	+ 6	+ 8	N.R. 6 cc.	+ 2	− 9	−11
E.S. 6 cc.	− 8	− 6	+ 2	J.T. 5 cc.	+ 2	− 2	− 4
C.S. 5 cc.	−11	− 5	+ 6	P.B. 4 cc.	+ 8	−10	−18
H.B. 4 cc.	− 8	0	+ 8	W.H. 3 cc.	− 2	−11	− 9
				S.H. 3 cc.	0	− 5	− 5
				J.B. 4 cc.	−13	−13	0

The remaining 18 subjects had a basal metabolic rate of plus or minus 15 per cent or more either before or after marihuana was administered. Of these there was a rise in 14 and a fall in 4 following the ingestion of marihuana but in only 4 of these subjects was the rise significant, the rates being +30, +32, +18, and +25, after doses of 20, 2, 8, and 6 cc. respectively. The figures for this group are shown in Table 12.

The control figures are lower than those commonly reported. Of the 61 subjects, the rate in 11 was on the plus side, in 38 on the minus side within a range of +9 and −15 per cent, while for 4 it was 0. In 8 the rate was between −16 and −23 per cent. It is possible that prison life is conducive to a lowering of metabolic processes but our study is too limited to allow any generalization.

TABLE 12

Metabolic rates (in per cent) outside a range of from +9 to −13 per cent

Dose	Without Marihuana	Under Marihuana	Difference	Dose	Without Marihuana	Under Marihuana	Difference
Users				*Users*			
J.N. 13 cc.	−20	−17	+ 3	C.B. 11 cc.	− 7	−18	−11
T.R. 13 cc.	−17	− 8	+ 9	J.B. 5 cc.	− 2	−15	−13
B.W. 8 cc.	−22	−14	+ 8	J.K. 5 cc.	− 9	−17	− 8
J.P. 8 cc.	−15	− 4	+11				
F.G. 8 cc.	−12	+18	+30				
H.A. 8 cc.	−17	− 4	+13				
V.L. 6 cc.	+ 9	+25	+16				
W.R. 4 cc.	−17	−13	+ 4				
R.G. 2 cc.	+ 4	+32	+28				
E.S. 2 cc.	−23	−19	+ 4				
J.T. 2 cc.	−15	−12	+ 3				
Non-users				*Non-users*			
H.B. 20 cc.	+ 2	+30	+28	C.C. 3 cc.	−19	−23	− 4
J.G. 3 cc.	−15	−14	+ 1				
W.D. 3 cc.	−16	−14	+ 2				

From the figures shown, it may be concluded that in the majority of subjects, marihuana caused no appreciable change in metabolic rate, although in those having an initially low rate, there was usually a rise. What changes occurred had no relationship to marihuana dosage, and there was no distinction between users and non-users.

Vital Capacity

Along with the determination of the basal metabolic rate, the measurement of vital capacity was made on 66 subjects before and after marihuana was administered. There was a decrease in 41, an increase in 11, and no change in 14. Such changes as occurred were insignificant. The average vital capacity during the control period was 3.6 liters (range 2.3—5.1); after marihuana 3.5 liters (range 2.1—4.9).

SUMMARY

The most consistent effect of marihuana observed in this division of the study was an increase in pulse rate which began shortly after the taking of the drug, reached a peak in about two hours, and gradually disappeared. In a few instances a temporary sinus tachycardia or sinus bradycardia was noted, but except for these there were no abnormalities in rhythm. The increase in pulse rate was usually accompanied by a rise in blood pressure.

There was in general an increase in the blood sugar level and in the basal metabolic rate, quite marked in some subjects, but in the majority the levels reached did not exceed the high normal limits.

An increase in the frequency of urination was often observed. There was, however, no appreciable increase in the total amount of urine passed during the drug action.

Hunger and an increase in appetite, particularly for sweets, was noted in the majority of the subjects, and the taking of candy or sweetened drinks brought down a "too high" effect of the drug. Nausea and vomiting occurred in a number of instances, diarrhea only during psychotic episodes.

On the other hand, the blood showed no changes in cell count, hemoglobin per cent, or the urea nitrogen, calcium and phosphorus figures. The figures for the circulation rate and vital capacity and the results of the phenolsulfonphthalein test for kidney function and the bromsulfalein test for liver function were not different from those of the control period. The electrocardiograms showed no abnormalities which could be attributed to a direct action on the heart. In the few observations on gastric motility and secretion no evidence of marihuana action on these functions was obtained.

The positive results observed, increase in pulse rate and blood pressure, increase in blood sugar and metabolic rate, urge to urinate, increased appetite, nausea and vomiting, and diarrhea, were not intensified by an increase in dosage, for they could occur in an equal degree after the administration of any of the effective doses within the range used. All the effects described are known to be expressions of forms of cerebral excitation, the impulses from this being transmitted through the autonomic system. The alterations in the functions of the organs studied come from the effects of the drug on the central nervous system and are proportional to these effects. A direct action on the organs themselves was not seen.

Psychological Aspects

PSYCHOPHYSICAL AND OTHER FUNCTIONS

ROBERT S. MORROW, PH.D.

In this phase of the study an effort was made to determine the effect of marihuana on various psychomotor and some special mental abilities. Appraisal of these effects was made wherever possible through the use of standardized tests. A number of different tests were originally tried under varying experimental conditions on the group of 5 volunteer subjects who had never before taken marihuana. Only those tests were retained which, in the course of this preliminary investigation, demonstrated the greatest potentialities. With the tests finally selected it was hoped to measure the effect of marihuana on the following functions.

Functions and Capacities Tested

STATIC EQUILIBRIUM

This was measured by means of the Miles Ataxiameter which is an instrument for recording body sway. The subject remains stationary in the ataxiameter with his hands at his sides and his feet together while a system of pulleys attached to a helmet on his head records the direction and degree of movement. The subject's score is the cumulative sway in all directions measured in millimeters. This test was applied to each subject for two minutes with his eyes open and two minutes with his eyes closed. Each trial was followed by a rest period of five minutes.

HAND STEADINESS

Hand steadiness was measured by means of the Whipple Steadiness Tester which consists of a metal disk with a hole 3/16 of an inch in diameter, connected in series with dry cells, an electric counter, and a stylus. The subject was instructed to hold the stylus in the hole for two minutes without touching the metal sides. Each contact with the side of the hole was recorded and the total number of contacts gave an index of unsteadiness of hand.

Speed of Tapping

Speed of tapping was measured in somewhat the same manner as was hand steadiness. The Whipple Apparatus was used, the tapping board replacing the steadiness disk and a thicker and heavier stylus replacing the steadiness stylus. The subject tapped repeatedly on the metal plate for two minutes and the total number of taps was recorded on the counter, thereby giving a measure of motor speed.

Strength of Grip

The Collins Dynamometer was used to measure the subject's strength of grip. Three trials were made for each hand and the scores averaged.

Simple and Complex Hand and Foot Reaction Time

Special apparatus was constructed to measure simple and complex hand and foot reaction time. To measure simple hand reaction time, the subject was instructed to press down on a telegraph key and 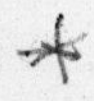 remove his hand as quickly as possible when a red light appeared on the board which stood directly before him. A Cenco counter recorded the reaction time, that is, the time which elapsed between the presentation of the stimulus and the response.

For the measurement of simple foot reaction time, the subject pressed down on a pedal with his foot, removing it as quickly as possible when the red light appeared.

For the measurement of complex (choice or discrimination) hand and foot reaction time either a red or a blue light served as a stimulus. The subject had no advance knowledge as to which color light would appear. For measuring the response with the hand, the subject pressed down on the telegraph key with the right hand and, at the sight of the red light, moved the peg from the red compartment into the center (neutral) compartment with the left hand, then removed the right hand from the key; at the appearance of the blue light, he moved the peg from the blue to the neutral compartment. For measuring complex foot reaction time, the procedure was similar to that for estimating the hand reaction time except that the right foot and the pedal were substituted for the right hand and the telegraph key.

Each subject made fifteen trials for each of the four variations.

Musical Aptitude

Musical aptitude was determined by means of the Kwalwasser-Dykema Music Tests. The eight tests administered were the tonal memory test, the quality discrimination test, the intensity discrimination test, the tonal movement test, the time discrimination test, the rhythm discrimination test, the pitch discrimination test, and the melodic taste test. The sum of the scores for these separate tests was used to give a total score for musical aptitude.

Auditory Acuity

By means of the Galton Whistle, the subjects' limits of auditory acuity were gauged for both ascending and descending frequencies. The final score was the average of the results of three trials in each direction.

Perception of Time

An attempt was made to appraise the subject's facility in estimating time by asking him to state when, after a given signal, he thought the following intervals had elapsed,—fifteen seconds, one minute, and five minutes. Several trials were given for each time interval and the average of the results of the trials was taken as the final score.

Perception of Length

Subjects were asked to estimate the length of lines which were 3 inches, 5 inches, and 8 inches in length and to draw lines of 3 inches and 7 inches.

The Subjects

Fifty-four subjects were used in this part of the experiment, 36 marihuana users and 18 non-users. The two groups were equated approximately for the following factors: age, height, weight, years of formal education, and number of arrests. The age range for the user group was from 21 to 45 years with 27.9 years as an average; the age range for the non-user group was from 22 to 43 years with 29.8 years as an average. The range in height for the users was from 54 to 75 inches with a mean of 67.5 inches; for the non-users the range was from 60 to 71 inches with a mean of 66.8 inches. Range in weight for the users was from 123 to 178 pounds with 151.3 pounds as the mean, for the non-users from 115 to 180 pounds with 149.5 pounds as the mean. The schooling of the user group ranged from no education at all to 10 years with a mean of 7.1 years; that of the non-users varied from 6 to 12 years with a mean of 8.3 years. As regards the number of arrests, the range for the users was from 1 to 20 with a mean of 5.1 and for the non-users from 1 to 15 with a mean of 5.3.

The two groups differed radically with respect to race. Of the 36 marihuana users, 11 (31 per cent) were white, 18 (50 per cent) were Negroes, and 7 (19 per cent) were Puerto Ricans. Of the 18 non-users, 12 (67 per cent) were white, 6 (33 per cent) were Negroes, and none were Puerto Rican.

In addition, the user group was analyzed with respect to the age when the marihuana habit was begun, the duration of the habit, the number of marihuana cigarettes generally smoked per day, and the period of deprivation. The variation of the habit as already described for the entire group of users applies to the 36 subjects studied here.

Procedure

The tests were first administered to the subjects before they had taken marihuana, then about a week later when they were under the influence of 2 cc. of marihuana, and finally another week later after 5 cc.* of marihuana had been administered. On each occasion the psychomotor tests for static equilibrium, hand steadiness, tapping, strength of grip, and reaction time were repeated at hourly intervals for eight successive hours in order that the time-effects of marihuana might be determined.** The other tests, that is, those measuring musical ability, auditory acuity, visual memory, and perception of time and length were given to the subjects while in the undrugged condition and from three to four hours after the drug had been administered. The music tests were given under normal conditions and after 5 cc. of marihuana had been administered, but not under a 2 cc. dosage.

* A dose of 5 cc. of marihuana proved "too much" for many of the non-user subjects in the sense that ingestion of this amount was often followed by nausea and general symptoms of malaise which interfered with further testing. For this reason the higher dose for non-users was sometimes reduced to 3 cc. or 4 cc. In all, only 6 of the non-user subjects took the 5 cc. dose. Accordingly, although the higher dosage is referred to as 5 cc. it should be noted that the actual amount used varied from 3 cc. to 5 cc.

** The scores for the first 25 users and 6 non-users were obtained every half hour but, since there was little difference between the half-hourly and hourly results it was decided to record hourly scores only, except for the first half hour.

In almost all instances the marihuana was given in the morning shortly after breakfast and generally after a day when no drug had been taken in order that "hangover" effects might be avoided. For the most part the subjects rested and did little or nothing except the prescribed tests on days when marihuana was taken.

The equilibrium, steadiness, tapping and strength of grip tests were given together on one day and the different forms of the reaction-time test on another day. Ordinarily four or five days elapsed between retests.

In addition to being tested after standard doses of the marihuana concentrate had been ingested, 11 users and 9 non-users were tested after smoking marihuana cigarettes.* The cigarettes weighed from 4 to 8 grains each. Most of the subjects smoked five cigarettes; two non-users smoked only three, and one non-user smoked four. The tests with cigarettes were given at quarter-hour, half-hour and hour intervals.

Findings

Static Equilibrium

Table 13 gives the averages of the scores of the 36 marihuana users and 18 non-users as tested on the Miles Ataxiameter prior to and after the ingestion of marihuana. In this and the subsequent tables all measures of variation have been omitted; however, the calculations were done and are available. In general, it was found that the variability of the subjects on most of the tests was considerable; for example, the scores on the first swaymeter trial for the subjects with eyes open ranged from 436 mm. to 1836 mm. and with eyes closed from 728 mm. to 2051 mm. Although the variation in performance was considerable it was not so large as to make unreliable the differences observed between the subjects in the drugged and the undrugged conditions. In the case of most of the tests the critical ratios were significant.

* A short experiment in which placebos were employed was also tried on these subjects. An attempt was made to have the placebos simulate the marihuana as much as possible but unfortunately the placebo pills had a distinctive taste which rendered them easily identifiable. The subjects referred to them as the "licorice" pills or the "blanks." While the experiment was completed and resulted in some interesting findings, the factors which might have invalidated the results were so serious that these experiments are not reported at this time.

TABLE 13

Effect of marihuana on static equilibrium as measured by the Miles Ataxiameter.

Time (in hours) after administration of marihuana	Eyes open						Eyes closed					
	Average sway of 36 users (in millimeters)			Average sway of 18 non-users (in millimeters)			Average sway of 36 users (in millimeters)			Average sway of 18 non-users (in millimeters)		
	Marihuana dosage			Marihuana dosage			Marihuana dosage			Marihuana dosage		
	0 cc.	2 cc.	5 cc.	0 cc.	2 cc.	3-5 cc.	0 cc.	2 cc.	5 cc.	0 cc.	2 cc.	3-5 cc.
1st trial.......	891			881			1197			1237		
½	858*	823*	808*	815†	826†	842†	1131*	1095*	1119*	1180†	1192†	1294†
1	833	850	983	849	899	1146	1148	1166	1301	1207	1270	1648
2	833	928	1167	842	985	1462	1122	1323	1560	1216	1544	2127
3	825	1015	1418	812	1446	1833	1145	1391	1840	1203	2042	2272
4	817	1039	1674	839	1636	2011	1114	1421	2028	1182	2329	2635
5	810	957	1433	822	1417	1960	1113	1319	1704	1152	1770	2352
6	813	889	1232	854	1241	1728	1110	1232	1508	1172	1494	2008
7	814	828	1066	850	1162	1436	1139	1137	1354	1157	1412	1836
8	816	830	972	821	958	1179	1114	1122	1248	1158	1288	1577

*First 25 subjects only.
†First 6 subjects only.

When marihuana was not administered (0 cc.), body equilibrium remained relatively unchanged over the eight-hour period. The discrepancy between the results of the first trial and those of subsequent trials is undoubtedly due to the failure of the subjects to become adjusted immediately to the experimental situation.

When 2 cc. of marihuana was administered to the users (eyes open) unsteadiness became slightly greater at the end of the second hour following ingestion and increased until it reached its highest point after four hours. It then receded gradually until the seventh hour when the pre-marihuana condition was regained. After the administration of 5 cc. (eyes open), the unsteadiness began at the first hour, increased more rapidly and reached its maximum also at the end of four hours, then receded but did not return to the level of the undrugged performance after eight hours. As far as the user is concerned, therefore, static equilibrium was adversely affected by 27 per cent when the 2 cc. and no-marihuana conditions are compared at the fourth-hour periods and by 105 per cent when the 5 cc. and no-marihuana conditions are compared at the fourth-hour periods.

As for the non-user tested with his eyes open, the effect of the 2 cc. dose was apparent earlier and was more intense than it was on the user, beginning during the first hour, reaching a higher peak at the end of four hours, and not returning to pre-marihuana levels at the end of eight hours. The pattern of the performance under 3 to 5 cc. of marihuana was in general the same as that under the 2 cc. dosage, but under the larger dose unsteadiness was far greater. For the non-user, static equilibrium was affected adversely by 95 per cent and 140 per cent by respective doses of 2 cc. and 5 cc. of marihuana.

When the marihuana users were tested for static equilibrium with their eyes closed, the general performance was very much like that which occurred when the eyes were open. A comparison of the results of the fourth-hour tests shows that the unsteadiness was increased by 28 per cent and 82 per cent under doses of 2 cc. and 5 cc. of marihuana respectively.

For the non-users also, unsteadiness increased for four hours after ingestion, the percentage of increase over the normal at the fourth-hour interval being 97 under 2 cc. and 123 under 5 cc. of marihuana.

Analysis of the data with regard to forward and backward motions as well as those along the right and left axes showed that there was no greater swaying in one direction than in any other.

Hand Steadiness

Table 14 gives the results of the tests on hand steadiness for both the users and the non-users under normal conditions and after they had ingested varying doses of marihuana. Here again it should be stated that variations in individual performance were great, the range in the first trial being from 0 to 136 contacts, so that the means are valid for interpretation of performance in relative but not absolute terms.

TABLE 14

Effect of marihuana on hand steadiness (right hand) as measured by the Whipple Steadiness Board

Time (in hours) after administration	Average number of contacts made by 36 users			Average number of contacts made by 18 non-users		
	Marihuana Dosage			Marihuana Dosage		
	0 cc.	2 cc.	5 cc.	0 cc.	2 cc.	3-5 cc.
1st trial.....	28.5			30.3		
½	21.8*	19.1*	17.8*	36.1†	24.2†	23.7†
1	22.3	21.7	25.3	24.5	28.5	33.0
2	21.6	24.3	40.4	21.2	37.4	66.2
3	23.6	33.5	53.9	19.3	63.4	74.3
4	20.4	36.0	59.8	18.2	62.7	84.6
5	18.4	31.4	46.2	16.7	49.4	64.0
6	18.1	26.2	39.3	17.0	43.6	54.1
7	18.7	21.4	31.7	15.9	45.4	49.0
8	16.6	18.7	28.0	16.7	25.1	37.3

*First 25 subjects only.
†First 6 subjects only.

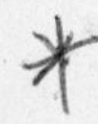

Unsteadiness of hand, like unsteadiness of equilibrium, was increased by the ingestion of marihuana, and the maximum effect again occurred about four hours after ingestion of the drug. The dosage of 5 cc. had a greater effect than that of 2 cc. and the non-users were affected to a greater degree than were the users. A comparison of the results of the fourth-hour tests reveals that under doses of 2 cc. and 5 cc. of marihuana unsteadiness of hand increased by 76 per cent and 193 per cent respectively for the user and by 245 per cent and 365 per cent* respectively for the non-user.

* The large increase in hand unsteadiness cannot be interpreted as representing an increased tremor of the hand alone. The actual number of "contacts" was the result of a number of factors, some of which, like the subjects' increased drowsiness and general indifference, were not directly related to hand tremor. Further experiments would be necessary to permit the drawing of any inferences as regards neurological origin and significance of this unsteadiness.

Strength of Grip

The changes in the strength of grip following the ingestion of marihuana were generally negligible in the case of both user and non-user. For the user there were average decreases of only 1 per cent and 9 per cent four hours after the ingestion of 2 cc. and 5 cc. of marihuana respectively as compared to the fourth-hour level under normal conditions, while for the non-users these decreases were 7 per cent and 10 per cent. The detailed findings are given in Table 15.

Table 15

Effect of marihuana on strength of grip as measured by the Collins Dynanometer

Time (in hours) after administration	Average strength (measured in kilograms) of 36 users			Average strength (measured in kilograms) of 18 non-users		
	Marihuana dosage			Marihuana dosage		
	0 cc.	2 cc.	5 cc.	0 cc.	2 cc.	3-5 cc.
1st trial.....	50.5			47.3		
½	50.7*	51.8*	51.9*	48.8†	48.9†	47.8†
1	51.3	51.6	51.0	47.5	47.1	47.8
2	51.1	50.7	49.4	49.2	48.1	46.3
3	51.6	51.0	48.4	48.6	46.0	45.8
4	51.1	50.6	46.7	48.5	45.1	43.7
5	51.1	50.5	47.6	48.1	44.9	45.1
6	51.2	50.5	47.3	48.1	45.3	45.0
7	51.3	51.0	49.7	47.7	46.8	46.1
8	51.7	51.0	49.3	48.3	46.9	46.9

*First 25 subjects only.
†First 6 subjects only.

Speed of Tapping

By and large it appears that speed of tapping was only slightly decreased by the ingestion of marihuana. At the fourth-hour interval the decreases in average speed under 2 cc. and 5 cc. of marihuana as compared with the performance under normal conditions were respectively 3 per cent and 6 per cent for the users and 7 per cent and 4 per cent for the non-users.

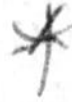

Reaction Time

Simple hand and foot reaction times were not affected by the ingestion of marihuana regardless of the amount of the drug taken and of the time elapsing after its administration. For the simple

hand reaction time the fourth-hour means were .11 seconds (no marihuana), .11 seconds (2 cc.), and .12 seconds (5 cc.) for the user, and .11 seconds in all three instances for the non-user. For simple foot reaction time the fourth-hour means were .16 seconds (no marihuana), .17 seconds (2 cc.), and .18 seconds (5 cc.) for the user and .16 seconds (no marihuana), .17 seconds (2 cc.), and .17 seconds (5 cc.) for the non-user.

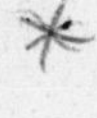

However, the ingestion of marihuana did affect complex hand and foot reaction time (Table 16) except in the case of the user after the ingestion of 2 cc. of the drug. After the administration of 5 cc. the user showed an impairment of 20 per cent in complex hand reaction time and 18 per cent in complex foot reaction time if the tests at the fourth-hour intervals are compared.

The complex hand and foot reaction times of the non-user were affected by marihuana administered in doses of either 2 cc. or 5 cc. At the fourth-hour testing periods there was a falling off of 28 per cent and 43 per cent in hand reaction time and 28 per cent and 38 per cent in foot reaction time under respective doses of 2 cc. and 5 cc. of marihuana.

Musical Ability and Auditory Acuity

The ingestion of marihuana (5 cc.) produced little or no effect on the subjects' scores on the musical ability tests. This applied to both the 30 users and the 12 non-users who were tested. The results from these tests would seem to indicate that the use of marihuana does not improve musical ability, at least insofar as non-musicians are concerned.

The results with the Galton Whistle paralleled generally those of the music tests. On the whole, the acuity of pitch perception of both user and non-user was not changed by the ingestion of marihuana.

Estimation of Time and Length

The data obtained from the tests used to measure these functions are given in Tables 17 and 18. As regards the estimation of time, the results at first glance might seem to corroborate statements found in the literature that time drags for persons under the influence of marihuana, but, on the other hand, they also indicate that it passed just as slowly for the subjects before the ingestion of the drug. According to our objective measurements, marihuana did not affect the ability of the subjects to estimate relatively short time intervals.

TABLE 16

Effect of marihuana on complex hand and foot reaction times

Time (in hours) after administration	Hand						Foot					
	Average reaction time of 36 users (in seconds)			Average reaction time of 18 non-users (in seconds)			Average reaction time of 36 users (in seconds)			Average reaction time of 18 non-users (in seconds)		
	Marihuana dosage			Marihuana dosage			Marihuana dosage			Marihuana dosage		
	0 cc.	2 cc.	5 cc.	0 cc.	2 cc.	3-5 cc.	0 cc.	2 cc.	5 cc.	0 cc.	2 cc.	3-5 cc.
1st trial	1.29			1.40			1.28			1.35		
½	1.19*	1.04*	.97*	1.22†	1.12†	1.02†	1.16*	1.04*	.98*	1.26†	1.08†	.96†
1	1.15	1.02	.98	1.22	1.06	1.03	1.12	1.01	1.00	1.22	1.05	1.04
2	1.11	.98	1.02	1.12	1.10	1.16	1.04	.98	1.03	1.13	1.09	1.10
3	1.02	.99	1.14	1.03	1.19	1.41	1.02	.99	1.13	1.06	1.24	1.40
4	.99	.99	1.19	1.01	1.29	1.45	1.00	.99	1.18	1.02	1.31	1.41
5	.96	.96	1.07	.98	1.18	1.26	.96	.97	1.09	1.01	1.15	1.28
6	.93	.95	1.01	.96	1.08	1.12	.94	.93	1.03	.98	1.09	1.12
7	.91	.92	.97	.93	1.01	1.05	.94	.92	.98	.99	1.03	1.04
8	.92	.93	.95	.93	.97	.96	.93	.92	.96	.96	.98	1.00

*First 25 subjects only.
†First 6 subjects only.

TABLE 17

Influence of marihuana on estimation of time

Dose	Average estimate made of		
	15 seconds (in seconds)	60 seconds (in seconds)	5 minutes (in minutes)
31 *Users*			
No drug	9.0	30.9	2.52
2 cc	8.7	31.7	2.75
5 cc	8.9	30.6	2.75
10 *Non-users*			
No drug	8.8	33.5	3.07
2 cc	8.5	31.0	2.93
5 cc	8.3	30.5	2.89

TABLE 18

Influence of marihuana on estimation of length

Dose	Average estimate (in inches) made of			Average line (in inches) drawn for	
	3 inches	5 inches	8 inches	3 inches	7 inches
31 *Users*					
No drug	3.0	4.8	8.1	3.0	6.3
2 cc	2.9	5.0	8.1	3.1	6.3
5 cc	3.0	4.9	8.1	3.1	6.3
11 *Non-users*					
No drug	3.3	5.2	8.6	2.9	6.0
2 cc	3.2	5.5	8.7	3.0	6.7
5 cc	3.5	5.6	8.5	2.8	6.6

However, if subjective criteria are of any value, it is interesting to note that many subjects reported that time passed very slowly for them when they were required to do something while under the influence of marihuana. In some instances a performance which took only two minutes (for example, standing under an ataxiameter) appeared to the subject to take a half-hour.

The results from the experiments in which subjects were asked to estimate the length of 3-, 5-, and 8-inch lines and to draw lines 3 inches and 7 inches long show that, for short lengths at least, the drug caused no observable deterioration in such type of judgment.

Tests with Cigarettes

Part of the experiment described above was repeated on 11 users and 9 non-users after they had smoked marihuana cigarettes. The users smoked five cigarettes in from one-half to one and a quarter hours and the non-users from three to five cigarettes in from one quarter to one and a quarter hours.

The effects of smoking marihuana on static equilibrium and hand steadiness are shown in Table 19. They were very similar to those observed after the ingestion of marihuana in pill form, except that they occurred much sooner. The quicker action of the marihuana in cigarette form necessitated appraisal of the drug action at much shorter intervals so that instead of taking readings at every hour the first few readings were taken at fifteen-minute intervals. The action was so rapid that when the subject was tested a quarter of an hour after he had smoked a cigarette there was already impairment in functioning. In body steadiness and hand steadiness this impairment amounted to as much as 75 per cent. After this quarter-hour peak there was a progressive lessening of the impairment until the end of the third hour when the effect of the cigarette was no longer evident.

This held true for those functions which the marihuana taken in pill form affected adversely to a marked degree. In the case of functions like strength of grip where the marihuana concentrate had little effect there was likewise no indication of adverse effect when cigarettes were used.

It should be noted that these results represent trends rather than invariable findings. It appears that the tendency of the non-user to be affected more adversely than the user was not as consistent when marihuana cigarettes were smoked as it was when the marihuana was ingested in pill form. The initial effect lasted longer for the user because, being accustomed to using marihuana he smoked more effectively and absorbed more of the drug than did the non-user.

Effect of Marihuana on Females

Five women prisoners from the House of Detention were studied to see if there were any important differences between the reactions of women and those of men to marihuana. Four of the 5 women were drug addicts who used marihuana occasionally and the fifth was an habitual marihuana user. Three were white and 2, includ-

TABLE 19

Effect of marihuana cigarettes on static equilibrium and hand steadiness

Time (in hours) after smoking	Static equilibrium: Average sway (in millimeters)								Hand steadiness: Average number of contacts			
	Eyes open				Eyes closed							
	11 users		9 non-users		11 users		9 non-users		11 users		9 non-users	
	No. cigarettes 0	5	No. cigarettes 0	3-5	No. cigarettes 0	5	No. cigarettes 0	3-5	No. cigarettes 0*	5	No. cigarettes 0*	3-5
Immediately		1431		1683		2069		2545		58.8		68.2
¼		1460		1535		2081		2144		55.8		69.0
½		1379		1353		1693		1942		57.0		58.9
1	861	1183	816	1399	1163	1769	1173	1828	22.3	45.2	24.5	68.4
1½		1155		1268		1616		1606		33.4		51.8
2	844	1060	766	1144	1186	1570	1200	1476	21.6	42.2	21.2	39.7
3	908	901	762	1011	1178	1227	1112	1289	23.6	27.2	19.3	23.8

*The figures here do not represent the averages of the 11 users and 9 non-users reported but the means for the entire group as given in Table 2. This may introduce some error in absolute values but the impairment in hand steadiness during and immediately after smoking marihuana is so great that the general conclusions would remain warranted.

TABLE 20

Effect of marihuana upon five women

Time (in hours) after administration	Static equilibrium						Hand steadiness			Strength of grip		
	(Eyes open)			(Eyes closed)								
	Average sway (in mm.)			Average sway (in mm.)			Average number of contacts			Average grip (in Kg.)		
	Marihuana dosage			Marihuana dosage			Marihuana dosage			Marihuana dosage		
	0 cc.	2 cc.	3-5 cc.	0 cc.	2 cc.	3-5 cc.	0 cc.	2 cc.	3-5 cc.	0 cc.	2 cc.	3-5 cc.
1	801	797	1116	1048	967	1506	30.6	25.4	65.2	29.2	30.2	28.9
2	769	873	1304	975	1047	1628	31.0	37.6	95.4	30.1	30.7	28.4
3	790	957	1308	1087	1142	1495	26.8	42.8	92.4	29.7	29.3	27.0
4	821	1033	1155	976	1113	1638	30.6	43.4	80.8	30.2	29.4	24.5
5	785	1010	1208	978	1052	1378	30.2	43.4	85.6	30.0	29.1	23.9
6	793	964	1020	909	1069	1157	23.4	33.2	59.0	29.4	30.0	25.1
7	856	845	907	982	992	1206	29.2	34.8	44.2	29.0	29.6	26.1
8	798	810	897	928	967	1107	28.4	27.2	31.8	29.7	30.6	25.7

ing the marihuana user, were Negroes. Their age range was from 28 to 35 years with 30.5 years as the average.

The women were given the majority of the tests which the men took and under the same conditions. In the case of one subject 3 cc. of marihuana was substituted for the 5 cc. dose.

The scores made by the women (see Table 20), though showing marked variation in individual cases owing to the poor sampling of the group, nevertheless followed the same general trends as those made by the men. However, it should be noted that in the case of the women under higher doses of marihuana, the effects of the drug frequently reached their maximum at an earlier hour and in some instances tended to taper off more abruptly. There were some other indications as regards quantitative differences in the performance of men and women under the influence of marihuana but the number of women subjects was too small to permit any further conclusions to be drawn.

As regards some of the supplementary tests such as musical ability and line and time perception, the general results were similar to those obtained from the experiments with male subjects.

Summary and Conclusions

1. The effect of marihuana on the psychomotor functions depends primarily on the complexity of the function tested. Simpler functions like speed of tapping and simple reaction time are affected only slightly by large doses (5 cc.) and negligibly, if at all, by smaller doses (2 cc.). On the other hand, the more complex functions like static equilibrium, hand steadiness, and complex reaction time may be affected adversely to a considerable degree by the administration of both large and small doses of marihuana.

2. The function most severely affected is body steadiness and hand steadiness. The ataxia is general in all directions rather than predominant in any particular axis.

3. The effects produced by larger doses (5 cc.) are systematically, though not necessarily proportionately, greater than those brought about by small doses.

4. The time required by the drug to exert its maximum effect varies somewhat with the function and size of dose, but, on the whole, time curves for both functions and dosages have similarity of form. The effect of the drug begins from one to two hours after

ingestion and reaches its peak at the fourth hour, after which it declines so that by the end of the eighth hour most of it is dissipated.

5. When marihuana is taken in cigarette form the psychomotor effects are similar in character and trend to those observed after the ingestion of the drug but they occur much sooner and taper off more quickly.

6. The effects seem to be essentially the same for women as for men, except that women are sometimes affected maximally at the second or third hour after the drug is administered. In women the return to the normal condition is in some instances quicker and more abrupt than it is in the men.

7. Non-users generally seem to be more affected by the drug when it is ingested than are users.

8. Auditory acuity is not affected by marihuana.

9. There is no evidence that musical ability, of non-musicians at least, is improved by marihuana.

10. The ability to estimate short periods of time and short linear distances is not measurably affected by the ingestion of marihuana.

INTELLECTUAL FUNCTIONING

Florence Halpern, M.A.

In this phase of the study investigation was directed primarily toward establishing the effect of marihuana on the subject's intellectual functioning. An attempt was made to determine what changes in mental ability occur under different amounts of the drug, what direction these changes take, when they are first measurable, and how long they persist.

Tests

Bellevue Adult Intelligence Test

This test was used to measure the general mental level of all the subjects. It was chosen in preference to other available scales because it is the only individual test of intelligence which has been standardized on an adult population, takes into account both verbal and performance abilities, and compares the individual with standards established for his particular age group. It consists of ten tests, five verbal and five performance. The verbal tests cover the fields of general information and general comprehension, draw on the individual's capacity for abstract reasoning and test his arithmetical ability and his rote memory. The performance tests also evaluate the subject's comprehension of social situations, but here the results are independent of language. There are also tests of the individual's ability to carry out a routine task, to organize parts into a meaningful whole, to distinguish between essential and unessential details, and to analyze and synthesize.

ARMY ALPHA (Bregman Revision, Forms A, B, 5, 7 and Bellevue Revision)

This is a group test first used in the United States Army in 1917 and 1918 when it was given to more than a million recruits. It consists of eight tests: test 1, a direction test which was not used in this study since the item does not appear on all forms; test 2, a test of arithmetical reasoning; test 3, a test of common sense in which the subject indicates which he considers the best of three possible responses to a given question; test 4, a modified vocabulary test; test 5, in which the subject must mentally reorganize disarranged sentences and then indicate whether the resultant statement is true or false; test 6, a test of numerical relations in which the subject must supply the last two numbers in a numerical series on the basis of the relationship between the first six numbers; test 7, a test of analogies in which the subject determines the relationship between two given words and then underlines one of four words which is related to a third word in the same way; and test 8, which on Forms A and B and on the Bellevue Revision is a test of general information in which the subject is given a choice of five answers to a question. On Forms 5 and 7, this test is a test of directions.

Because this test has five alternate forms which are roughly of equivalent difficulty it could be repeated many times within a short time interval. It was therefore used to establish a curve showing at what time following ingestion the marihuana has an effect on general intelligence and on individual higher mental processes.

PYLE'S DIGIT SYMBOL TEST

In this test each number from 1 through 9 is associated with a specific symbol, as, for example, number 1 is associated with a square and number 2 with an asterisk. The numbers and their associated symbols appear at the top of the sheet of paper. Below the sample are rows of symbols, five symbols to a row, followed by five blank squares. The subject is expected to fill in each square with the number associated with the respective symbol. With practice the association bond between the number and the symbol becomes stronger and the subject depends less and less on the model at the top of the sheet. He is therefore able to work faster and his learning rate is reflected in the increased number of squares filled.

Cancellation Test

The subject is required to cross out a specific geometric form wherever it appears on a sheet which is covered with rows of geometric figures. This measures the individual's capacity for carrying out a routine task.

Form Board Test

The measurement of the ability to manipulate concrete material in contrast to the verbal or abstract ability determined by the Army Alpha test required the introduction of certain form board tests. These were the Seguin Form Board, the Two Figure Board, the Casuist Board, the Five Figure Board, Healy A, Triangle Test, Diagonal Test, all administered and scored according to the Pintner-Patterson Performance Series. The Seguin Form Board has ten blocks of various geometric forms, to be put in their appropriate places as rapidly as possible. Three trials are given. The Two Figure Board has nine pieces which, when placed correctly, form a large cross and a large square. Time and the number of moves are recorded. The Casuist Board has twelve pieces which, when correctly placed, form three circles and an oval. Time and errors are recorded. The Five Figure Board has five geometrical figures which are formed by the correct placement of two or three pieces for each figure. Time and errors are recorded. Healy A has five small rectangular pieces which, when placed correctly, form a large rectangle. Time and the number of moves are recorded. The Triangle Test consists of four triangular pieces which are fitted together in a board. Time and errors are recorded. The Diagonal Test has five pieces of various shapes which must be fitted together in a rectangular frame. Time and moves are recorded.

Kohs Block Design Test

This is a performance test which is less a test of manual dexterity and more dependent on abstract intelligence than are the form board tests. It correlates more highly with intelligence than do most performance items and yet it is entirely independent of language. Therefore, the individual who cannot express himself well or who suffers from a language handicap is not penalized as he is on verbal scales.

The test consists of sixteen cubes each with a red, a white, a blue, a yellow, a red-and-white, and a blue-and-yellow side. A colored design which can be reproduced with the cubes is placed before the subject and he is expected to make it. Results are rated numerically, depending upon the time consumed in execution. In this experiment two sets of designs of equivalent difficulty were required; Designs IV, VI, and XIV were selected for one series and V, VII, and XII for the other.

Memory Tests

Although memory in itself cannot be considered a measure of intelligence, it is essential to any intelligent functioning and must therefore be included in any estimate of intelligence. Three aspects of memory, namely rote memory, the ability to recall presented objects, and visual memory were tested. The rote memory test requires the repetition of digits in forward and reverse order as given on the Bellevue Intelligence Test. Object memory was tested by exposing ten small objects for three seconds and recording the number of articles the subject was able to recall. Visual memory or the ability to reproduce designs after a ten-second exposure was estimated by using the designs and scoring technique from the Army Performance Test.

Procedure

The Bellevue Adult Intelligence Test

Each subject was given the Bellevue Adult Intelligence test within two or three days after his admission to the hospital and before any marihuana had been administered.

The Army Alpha, Pyle's Digit Symbol, and Cancellation Tests

These tests were given as group tests to a total of 20 subjects. The Army Alpha and Pyle's Digit Symbol tests were given every half-hour, beginning a half-hour after drug ingestion. The Army Alpha was continued for seven hours and Digit Symbol for five hours. The Cancellation test was given every hour for six hours, beginning one hour after drug administration. Eleven users and 9 non-users took the Army Alpha and the Digit Symbol tests, while 9 users and 11 non-users took the Cancellation test.

Tests 2 through 8 of the Army Alpha require twenty and a half minutes for actual performance while such preparations as the distribution of papers and the reading of directions consume almost ten minutes more, so that had the entire Alpha been given at each half-hourly session, the subjects would have gone from test to test with no intermittent rest period. For this reason the tests were divided and the following schedule arranged:

	First Day		*Second Day*
Test 2	5 minutes	Test 6	3 minutes
Test 3	1½ minutes	Test 7	3 minutes
Test 4	2* minutes	Test 8	4 minutes
Test 5	2 minutes	Cancellation	1½ minutes
Digit Symbol	2 minutes		
			11½ minutes
	12½ minutes		

Each subject took three test series, one without the drug, one with 2 cc. and one with 3, 4, 5, or 6 cc., depending on individual tolerance. A test series consisted of fourteen half-hourly sessions for the Alpha, ten half-hourly sessions for the Digit Symbol and seven hourly sessions for the Cancellation tests. Because of the time factor, a series required two days for its completion.

The halves of a series were given on successive days, and the different series a week apart. Thus for example, a subject might take his first test series with 2 cc. on Monday and Tuesday of one week; the following Monday and Tuesday the series would be repeated with the subject in a different drug state (no drug or 5 cc.); and a

* Although one and a half minutes is the usual time allotment for this test, two minutes were used for it in this study.

final series would be given the third week with the subject in still another drug condition.

An effort was made to obviate practice effect by giving the first test series to one third of the subjects without drug, to one third with 2 cc., and to one third with 3, 4, or 5 cc. However, because of the necessity of increasing dosage gradually this ideal presentation was not actually obtained. The following gives the amount of drug administered to users and non-users at each test series.

Users No. of cases	Size of Dose (in cc.)	*Non-Users* No. of cases	Size of Dose (in cc.)
3	0, 2, 5*	3	0, 2, 5
3	2, 5, 0	2	2, 5, 0
2	5, 0, 2	1	-, 5, 0***
1	5, 0, -**	2	2, 0, 5
2	5, 2, 0	1	2, 0, -****

1st Trial	2nd Trial	3rd Trial	1st Trial	2nd Trial	3rd Trial
0 cc. - 3	0 cc. - 3	0 cc. - 5	0 cc. - 3	0 cc. - 3	0 cc. - 3
2 cc. - 3	2 cc. - 5	2 cc. - 2	2 cc. - 5	2 cc. - 3	2 cc. - 0
5 cc. - 5	5 cc. - 3	5 cc. - 3	5 cc. - 0	5 cc. - 3	5 cc. - 5

Since the various forms of the Army Alpha are not absolutely equivalent in difficulty, their order of presentation for any one group had to be identical in each of the three drug states. However, for each of the three groups tested the order of presentation was different so that all the difficult forms did not come at the same interval, as is shown on the following page.

Kohs Block Design, Form Board and Memory Tests

Administration of these tests differed markedly from those discussed above in that no attempt was made to give them at regular successive time intervals. Rather, they formed part of a battery of individual tests given to various subjects under specific drug condi-

* 5 cc. is used to indicate large doses although the amount ranged from 3 cc. to 6 cc. depending on individual tolerance. In the non-user group no maximum dose for this test was more than 4 cc.

** Entered experiment too late to take more than two series.

*** Patient took initial series with 5 cc. but became so ill test was discontinued and only two subsequent series given.

**** Patient discharged from experiment before third series was given.

tions. For example, 5 cc. of marihuana would be ordered for a patient for 8:00 a.m., and testing began as soon thereafter as the patient appeared "high," the state of "highness" being judged by the subject's own statement, his pulse rate, the condition of his pupils and other physiological signs.

TIME	GROUP I	GROUP II	GROUP III
9:30	A	5	Bellevue
10:00	5	B	7
10:30	B	A	5
11:00	7	7	A
11:30	A	Bellevue	B
12:00	5	5	Bellevue
12:30	B	B	7
1:00	7	A	5
1:30	A	7	A
2:00	5	Bellevue	B
2:30	B	5	Bellevue
3:00	7	B	7
3:30	A	A	5
4:00	5	7	A

Kohs Block Design was given to each subject twice, once without the drug and once with 5 cc. The test was taken by a total of 21 subjects, 10 users and 11 non-users. Five users took the test first without the drug, 5 had their first trial with 5 cc. Of the non-user group 8 had their first trial without marihuana, 3 with 4 cc. The average time at which the test was given to the user group was three and a half hours after drug administration, with range from two to five and a half hours. For the non-user group, the average time of administration of the test was also three and a half hours after the drug was given, range two and a half to five and a half hours.

The two series of designs (one series being Designs IV, VI and XIV, the other V, VII and XII) were presented in such manner that half of the subjects were tested on one series and half on the other series while they were under the influence of marihuana. Thus any difference in degree of difficulty between the two sets of designs was cancelled out. The weighted scores given on the Arthur Point scale were used in evaluating the results.

Form Board tests were divided into three batteries, each battery consisting of the Seguin Form Board, one of the three larger boards

(Two Figure, Five Figure, or Casuist) and one of the three smaller boards. Various combinations of boards were used under various drug conditions in order to make the results as comparable as possible. The following indicates the number of times the various boards were used with different dosages of marihuana.

	0 cc.	2 cc.	5 cc.	TOTAL
Casuist	8	6	6	20
Two Figure	5	7	6	18
Five Figure	6	5	6	17
Diagonal	6	5	8	19
Triangle	7	4	9	20
Healy A	6	7	3	16

From the above it appears that Gwyn Triangle was used too often with 5 cc. and Healy A was not used often enough. Aside from the Triangle and the Healy A, the distribution of boards in different drug stages was such as to obviate any differences in degree of difficulty. Nineteen subjects, 10 users and 9 non-users, took this test. The results were scored for time and errors according to the Pintner-Patterson Performance series.

Memory tests. The first digit span test was always given before marihuana had been administered, since the Bellevue Scale was given each patient during the first two or three days of the study. The trials under 2 cc. and 5 cc. were alternated. In all, 28 subjects, 17 users and 11 non-users, took this test before and after the ingestion of marihuana. The final score equaled the number of digits recalled.

To test Object Memory, ten small articles such as a key, a ring, a pill box, and a crayon were placed on a flat, neutral surface and exposed for three seconds. An attempt was made to vary some of the articles at each presentation so that six or seven were the same and three or four were different. Twenty-six subjects, 11 users and 15 non-users, took this test. They were so divided that 10 of them took the test the first time without drug, 10 with 2 cc., and 6 with 5 cc.

To test Visual Memory, Army designs were given each subject three times, once prior to the administration of marihuana, once under 2 cc., and once under 5 cc. The test was given to a total of 28 subjects, 16 users and 12 non-users. Because there is no alternate form for this test, results were definitely influenced by practice. Here, therefore, more than with any other test, it became important to arrange the order of administration. The following indicates the dosage of marihuana at the first test.

	0 cc.	2 cc.	5 cc.
User	6	5	5
Non-User	5	4	3
TOTAL	11	9	8

It is obvious that the initial examination was given slightly more often when the subjects were not under the influence of the drug. Improvement derived from practice is therefore more of a factor in the tests which were performed under marihuana.

Findings

Bellevue Adult Intelligence Test

General Intelligence. The results of the Bellevue Adult Intelligence Test which was administered to 60 subjects, 40 users and 20 non-users, are shown in Table 21. As has been pointed out elsewhere, these findings indicate that both the user and the non-user groups may be classified as of average intelligence.

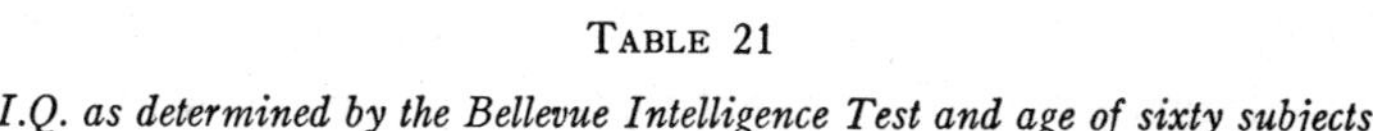

Table 21

I.Q. as determined by the Bellevue Intelligence Test and age of sixty subjects

Subjects	Age (in years)		Verbal I.Q.		Performance I.Q.		Total I.Q.	
	Average	Range	Average	Range	Average	Range	Average	Range
White								
13 Users....	27.7	21–34	105.6	79–125	105.7	78–129	106.1	77–124
15 Non-users	28.3	22–43	105.5	80–117	106.3	81–116	106.3	96–114
Negro								
19 Users....	27.8	22–45	93.1	77–118	93.2	67–112	92.6	70–112
5 Non-users	30.8	25–37	100.0	88–106	96.8	84–105	98.8	93–101
Puerto Rican								
8 Users....	29.0	24–34	91.5	73–100	92.2	74–108	91.0	72–100
Total								
40 Users....	28.5	21–45	96.9	73–125	97.1	74–129	96.7	70–124
20 Non-users	28.9	22–43	104.1	80–118	103.9	81–116	104.5	93–114

Mental Deterioration. Studies of mental deterioration due to toxic, organic or psychotic factors, as given in the literature, reveal that in such cases the subtest scores on the Bellevue Adult Intelligence Test show marked irregularity, depending upon the functions involved in the deteriorative process. As a group, the marihuana users tested show very even functioning, and what little irregularity occurred can be explained on the basis of language and racial factors.* From this we may conclude that the marihuana users had suffered no mental deterioration as a result of their use of the drug.

Army Alpha Test

Total Mental Functioning. The total scores obtained from this test at the successive testing periods are shown in Table 22. Those recorded before the administration of the drug give a picture like that seen in any learning curve, that is, there is a gradual increment in test scores at each testing interval, interspersed with plateau periods. Thus, without drug the test score for the second testing interval showed a 2 per cent gain over the initial score, the score for the third testing interval showed a 4 per cent gain over the initial score, and so on up to the last testing period when there was a 13 per cent gain over the initial test score.

Between two and a half and three hours after ingestion of 2 cc. of the drug there appeared to be a possible very slight falling off in mental ability. Otherwise the results paralleled the findings obtained in the undrugged condition except that toward the end of the day the increments were larger than those which occurred when the subjects were undrugged. This may be due to complications in the experimental procedure or may be an indication of accelerated mental functioning resulting from drug ingestion. This point is discussed more fully when the effect on different mental functions is considered.

Deleterious effects were apparent an hour after the ingestion of 5 cc. of marihuana. There was a 3 per cent drop from the initial score at this one-hour period and this first attainment is not surpassed until four and a half hours after drug ingestion. From the four-and-a-half-hour period on to the end of the testing there were gradual increments in score.

---

*The age factor does not affect the result since the groups were well equated in this respect (see page 67)

TABLE 22

Effect of marihuana on mental functioning as shown by total scores on Army Alpha Tests made by twenty subjects

Time after ingestion (in hours)	Measurements of total scores made by twenty subjects under doses of														
	0 cc.					2 cc.					5 cc.				
	Average	S.D.	Range	*Smoothed average	Change over initial score (in %)	Average	S.D.	Range	*Smoothed average	Change over initial score (in %)	Average	S.D.	Range	*Smoothed average	Change over initial score (in %)
½	107.1	43.97	20–179			89.5	36.17	32–167			114.3	35.47	61–181		
				108.1					92.4					113.5	
1	109.1	48.32	26–192			95.3	37.88	48–186			112.6	37.39	58–180		
				110.1	2				95.7	4				110.2	−3
1½	111.1	44.46	28–185			96.0	38.15	36–181			107.8	34.81	54–161		
				112.9	4				99.4	8				108.5	−4
2	114.6	47.28	34–188			102.8	37.54	28–179			109.1	36.82	50–163		
				111.7	3				99.4	8				107.8	−5
2½	108.7	44.91	39–186			95.9	36.57	33–176			106.5	34.79	52–158		
				112.7	4				96.3	4				110.8	−2
3	116.7	44.75	38–184			96.6	35.03	48–182			115.0	35.73	60–172		
				117.7	9				98.6	7				113.3	0
3½	118.7	43.09	41–193			100.5	35.65	46–186			111.6	38.62	52–165		
				118.8	10				100.9	9				113.0	0
4	118.8	41.34	49–184			101.3	35.25	56–185			114.3	39.15	57–174		
				120.1	11				102.5	11				117.1	3
4½	121.3	40.77	51–190			103.7	35.19	41–184			119.8	35.19	66–177		
				118.6	10				102.5	11				118.9	5
5	115.8	43.57	41–191			101.3	33.59	36–184			118.0	34.22	65–169		
				117.2	8				105.0	14				120.2	6
5½	118.5	41.44	36–188			108.7	31.67	52–180			122.4	36.02	61–179		
				121.2	12				111.0	20				122.0	7
6	123.8	39.57	53–194			113.3	34.49	61–190			121.6	38.90	59–180		
				123.6	14				114.7	24				122.9	8
6½	123.3	40.29	56–187			116.1	33.18	66–183			124.2	36.17	70–179		
				122.1	13				115.7	25				125.5	11
7	120.8	44.06	43–191			115.2	36.24	51–189			126.7	35.01	71–174		

*Smoothed average is obtained by averaging scores of successive intervals.

Different Mental Functions. A very elaborate study was made of the scores made on the subtest (Table 23). Some irregularities occurred even in the undrugged state, and these may be attributed primarily to chance factors, as, for example, the difference in difficulty of the various test forms. On the whole, the findings were in line with those which one would expect in any situation where constant repetition increases efficiency.

The effects of 2 cc. of marihuana on the different mental functions were variable. Tests involving number concepts gave clear-cut, consistent findings and revealed that impairment occurred an hour after the drug was taken and continued for from two and a half to three hours after ingestion. Results of other tests showed that there was little if any loss in ability, and some of them, especially those done toward the end of the day, showed gains which exceeded the ones made in the undrugged state. It is not possible on the basis of the present data to ascertain whether these large increments indicate that small amounts of the drug serve as stimulants in situations dependent primarily upon verbal facility or whether they are due to certain complications in the test technique. The former theory coincides with the increased verbosity noted on other tests as well as with the clinical impression, but the latter also cannot be overlooked. Further investigation of this point is definitely indicated.

The effect of the 5 cc. dosage on each function was in line with that reported for total scores, that is there was a falling off in efficiency one hour after the drug was taken and this impairment continued for anywhere from three and a half to six and a half hours after ingestion. Here too the scores on tests involving number concepts were most severely affected, recovery for them taking place from six to six and a half hours after drug administration.

Degree and Duration of Drug Effect. In general it may be stated that marihuana has a deleterious effect on mental functioning, the extent, time of onset, and duration of the impairment being related to the amount of drug taken.

The adverse effect of the 2 cc. dosage on global intelligence was slight (about 3 per cent to 4 per cent impairment in efficiency) and of short duration, occurring at about two and a half hours after ingestion and lasting little longer than a half-hour or an hour. Certain mental functions, especially those dealing with number concepts appear to have been affected much earlier than others, the effect on the number test scores being measurable as early as one

TABLE 23

Effect of marihuana on individual mental functions as shown by Army Alpha Subtests on twenty subjects

Time after ingestion (in hours)	Average increase (in per cent) over initial score* in subtests for																	
	Arithmetical reasoning			Common sense			Same-opposite			Mixed sentences			Numerical relations			Analogies		
	Dose 0 cc.	2 cc.	5 cc.	Dose 0 cc.	2 cc.	5 cc.	Dose 0 cc.	2 cc.	5 cc.	Dose 0 cc.	2 cc.	5 cc.	Dose 0 cc.	2 cc.	5 cc.	Dose 0 cc.	2 cc.	5 cc.
1¼	3	1	−5	−3	−6	−6	0	13	−1	3	2	−2	2	−1	−2	2	6	−1
1¾	5	0	−9	3	0	−6	5	22	2	7	11	1	3	−6	−5	7	11	−4
2¼	7	0	−9	7	7	−1	−3	14	−7	3	7	−3	6	−1	−5	7	13	−5
2¾	9	2	−5	13	13	6	−7	10	−9	4	1	−6	10	0	−5	5	13	−7
3¼	10	8	−3	16	13	7	3	13	−4	9	8	−1	11	1	−6	10	18	−3
3¾	9	5	−4	15	13	3	4	11	−4	13	13	0	11	5	−2	12	14	3
4¼	9	3	−4	17	16	9	5	12	−2	15	19	1	11	5	−4	16	15	11
4¾	12	5	−3	20	14	6	0	4	−1	6	15	4	13	8	−7	16	19	11
5¼	12	9	−2	20	19	15	−3	5	6	−1	13	−7	14	10	−6	12	18	10
5¾	12	9	−1	23	25	18	3	19	4	4	19	1	12	11	−4	18	31	14
6¼	12	10	1	19	29	21	1	26	−5	9	24	8	13	8	−4	25	41	17
6¾	12	11	1	23	30	20	−3	23	−4	13	32	8	13	10	10	24	41	22

*Using smoothed curve.

hour after ingestion and continuing until two and a half hours after ingestion. For other functions, in particular those involving verbal facility, the results were variable, in some instances showing no adverse effect and even a slight acceleration.

The effect of 5 cc. of marihuana on global intellectual functioning was apparent within an hour from the time the drug was taken and was operative until four and a half hours after ingestion. All mental functions showed this early impairment but for some of them recovery from the adverse effect was earlier than for others. Those most severely impaired from point of view of duration were the ones dealing with number concepts.

The testing program was continued for only seven hours after the drug was taken and, therefore, any estimate of the effect of marihuana after this time is purely a subjective one. However, both the subject and the examiner felt that the drug produced a "hang-over" which in most cases continued into the following day. The subject complained of being headachy, sleepy, and unable to work at his usual level, and the examiner also noted that the subject did not work as well or as quickly when called upon to do something on a day following marihuana ingestion.

The impairment reported here is not entirely representative of the maximum impairment which occurs under the influence of marihuana. Two opposing variables account for the results obtained in the drugged condition. One variable is practice effect which tends to increase test scores with each succeeding trial. The other variable, the drug, tends to lower test scores. In the earlier sessions there was evidence that the marihuana, especially when given in large doses, is the more potent force as seen by the continuing downward trend of the curve during the first few hours. In these earlier phases, in spite of repetition, results were lower with each succeeding trial, or if there was no actual loss, the increments made were never comparable to those made in the undrugged state. Three or four hours after drug administration there was a general trend towards rising scores. Some of this gain must be attributed to increased practice effect which was counteracting, in part at least, the deleterious effect of the marihuana. For this reason it is not certain that the drug was less effective at later points in the curve than it was at the moment of seemingly greatest impairment. This seems particularly plausible because, beginning with the third hour, the subject was no longer working on new tasks but was actually repeating identical tasks that he performed earlier in the day. Thus, at the third hour the test form used was the same as the one given at the initial session; at the end of the three-and-a-half-hour period the form was the same as the one-hour examination, and so on. What is shown in the curves is the effect of marihuana on intellectual tasks with which the subject has become very familiar. For practical purposes the test situation has the advantage of being comparable with daily living since the tasks performed in daily routine are usually relatively familiar ones.

Speed Versus Power. Intellectual impairment under the influence of marihuana resulted from a loss in both speed and efficiency. There was a slowing up in output indicated by the difference in the number of items done before and after the administration of the drug. On the whole the number of test items attempted tended to increase at each succeeding examination period even when the subject was under the influence of marihuana, but the percentage of increase in the drugged state practically never equaled that attained for the corresponding time interval when the subject had not ingested the drug. The findings for the number of items done in the drugged and undrugged condition follow very closely the findings in respect to the number of items correctly done. From this it may be concluded that under the influence of marihuana an individual functions less rapidly and also less efficiently than when he has had no drug.

Careful analysis of what causes the loss in efficiency reveals that certain factors not necessarily related to mental ability per se were accountable for the reduced scores in the drugged state. For example, under the influence of the drug the subject felt dizzy, had blurred vision, or exhibited other handicapping physiological disturbances. These impeded his efficiency in putting his answer on the correct line, or marking a cross in the right box. Men were observed running their fingers across the page in an effort to keep their place. On the other hand, much of the intellectual loss can be ascribed to an impairment in the thinking processes, and there seemed to be a general confusion of ideas and inability to maintain a fixed goal. Some subjects reported that the reason they accomplished so little was that, by the time they had finished reading a question, they no longer remembered what their purpose in reading it had been. Occasionally perseveration of a form of response specific to one test was found in a subsequent test. For example, some forms of the Same-Opposite test require the subject to mark the answer "S" or "O."

In a later test requiring a plus or minus response occasional irrelevant "S's" or "O's" appeared.

Comparison of the Effect of Marihuana on User and Non-User. When the group is divided into marihuana users and non-users certain interesting and suggestive differences are revealed (Table 24). Although the general findings for total intelligence scores for the two groups follow similar curves, the deleterious effects were not as great on the user as on the non-user. Thus under 2 cc. of marihuana the user showed no real intellectual impairment except for a very short interval beginning about two and a half hours after ingestion and lasting for an hour or an hour and a half. In contrast to this he made gains both at the beginning of the testing and toward the end of the day which exceeded those made in the undrugged state. The non-user who had ingested 2 cc. of marihuana showed a definite drop in score beginning about two and a half hours after ingestion, and for a period from one and a half to two and a half hours after this time he did not make increments comparable to those which he made in the undrugged state. Following this, during the last two hours of testing he, like the user, obtained scores which showed an acceleration not paralleled in the undrugged state.

TABLE 24

Comparison of the effect of marihuana on the mental functioning of users and non-users as shown by total scores made on Army Alpha Tests

Time after ingestion (in hours)	Per cent increase over initial score* made under doses of					
	0 cc.		2 cc.		5 cc.	
	11 users	9 non-users	11 users	9 non-users	11 users	9 non-users
1¼	−1	6	1	6	−3	− 3
1¾	1	8	7	9	−1	− 7
2¼	4	3	10	3	2	−12
2¾	4	4	9	−1	3	− 7
3¼	5	12	8	6	2	− 2
3¾	6	14	9	10	1	− 2
4¼	9	14	14	8	7	0
4¾	9	11	17	4	11	− 1
5¼	7	10	15	12	12	0
5¾	11	13	17	24	11	4
6¼	12	17	20	29	11	6
6¾	9	18	22	29	14	7

*Using smoothed averages.

Under 5 cc. of marihuana both the user and the non-user showed a 3 per cent loss in efficiency within an hour of the time that the drug was taken. Although recovery was slow for both groups, the user was less severely affected as is indicated by the fact that at the next testing interval his score was only 1 per cent below his initial score as compared with a 7 per cent loss on the part of the non-user. The disparity in the degree of impairment for the two groups continued for several hours. The more marked drug effect in the case of the non-user was further evidenced by the fact that the user showed recovery four or four and a half hours after ingestion (as measured by the time when his scores approach those made when in the undrugged state) while the non-user, even at the end of seven hours of testing, did not approximate his undrugged performances.

No simple explanation of this difference is available. The most probable reason seems to be that previous use of the drug in some way serves to ameliorate the anxiety and inevitable disorganization which the use of any drug may have on an individual who has never taken it before. Another explanation may lie in a possible physiological adaptation to the drug which, though not identical with tolerance in the ordinary pharmacological sense, seems to act in the same direction.

Variability. The results reported here are all in terms of averages. A study of individual scores indicates that there was marked variability in the effect of the drug on different subjects. In one case the drug action came early and soon disappeared. Another subject experienced no reaction until after he had eaten his lunch at which time a very definite effect was apparent. A third subject showed impairment late in the day when the drug effect on almost all the other subjects had worn off. There were some hardy souls who did not appear to be affected by even large quantities of marihuana, while a few (mainly non-users) became so ill that they could not continue with the examinations.

Pyle's Digit Symbol Test

Comparison of the results obtained on this test when the subject was in the undrugged condition and when he had had 2 cc. of marihuana reveals that small amounts of the drug did not interfere with his ability to carry out the appointed task (Table 25). In fact, as was noted above for certain other tests, the improvement in score at the end of two and a half or three hours was greater after the ingestion of 2 cc. of marihuana than it was when no drug had been administered, and at the end of the five-hour testing period there was a 32 per cent increase in score as against a 22 per cent increase in the undrugged condition.

TABLE 25

Effect of marihuana on learning ability as measured by Pyle's Digit Symbol Test

Time after ingestion (in hours)	Marihuana Dosage					
	0 cc. (20 subjects)		2 cc. (18 subjects)		4-5 cc. (19 subjects)	
	Average Score* (smoothed)	Increase over initial score (in %)	Average score* (smoothed)	Increase over initial score (in %)	Average score* (smoothed)	Increase over initial score (in %)
¾	78.6	—	60.8	—	75.4	—
1¼	82.8	5	63.8	5	77.5	3
1¾	85.9	9	66.3	9	77.7	3
2¼	88.4	12	71.1	17	78.6	4
2¾	91.9	17	75.5	24	79.0	5
3¼	92.6	18	73.9	22	80.6	7
3¾	92.9	18	74.9	23	85.2	13
4¼	93.7	19	78.1	28	91.3	21
4¾	95.7	22	80.3	32	95.8	27

*Score = number of right answers—number of wrong answers.

Under the influence of 5 cc. of marihuana, however, there was a decrease in ability occurring within an hour after the time the drug was administered. Although the scores show no actual loss as compared with the inital score, the increments did not equal those made in the undrugged condition until from four to four and a half hours after ingestion.

It may therefore be concluded that certain types of learning ability are not affected by small amounts (2 cc.) of marihuana, but are impaired when larger amounts (5 cc.) are ingested.

CANCELLING A GEOMETRIC FORM

The results of this test are shown in Table 26.

With 2 cc. of marihuana, there was a slight falling off in the subject's efficiency occurring about three hours after drug ingestion. At that time he was 3 per cent less efficient than he had been an hour previous. With 5 cc. of marihuana there was a slowing up in the subject's ability to carry out the appointed task which was apparent two hours after drug ingestion (and possibly earlier). At that time

TABLE 26

Effect of marihuana on the ability to carry out a routine task as measured by the cancelling of geometric figures by twenty subjects

Time after ingestion (in hours)	Marihuana Dosage					
	0 cc.		2 cc.		4-5 cc.	
	Average score*	Increase over initial score (in %)	Average score*	Increase over initial score (in %)	Average score*	Increase over initial score (in %)
1	59.2	—	50.5	—	52.1	—
2	65.0	10	56.5	12	54.4	4
3	65.9	11	55.1	9	55.2	6
4	67.2	14	57.0	13	54.9	5
5	66.5	12	58.3	15	57.9	11
6	74.0	25	62.3	23	64.8	24

*Score = number of right answers—number of wrong answers.

there was only a 4 per cent increment over his intial score as compared with a 10 per cent increment in the undrugged state and a 12 per cent increment when the 2 cc. dosage had been administered. He improved only slightly at the three- and four-hour testing interval, and only at the five-hour interval did he show an appreciable improvement.

Apparently, the carrying out of a simple routine task is adversely affected to a slight degree and for a short period of time as the result of the ingestion of 2 cc. of marihuana, while the ingestion of 5 cc. of the drug produces adverse effects which are more severe and more lasting.

PERFORMANCE TESTS

Seguin Form Board. For adults of average intelligence this test is primarily one involving speed of reaction time. The average time taken by the subjects when they were not under the influence of marihuana was 12.8 seconds. This was increased to 14.0 and 14.1 seconds under dosages of 2 cc. and 5 cc. respectively. Thus, ingestion of marihuana in 2 cc. and 5 cc. doses caused a 9 per cent delay in performance time.

Form Boards. The time scores for this test remained practically the same whether no drug, 2 cc. or 5 cc. of marihuana had been administered, the average scores in terms of mental age being respectively 11.7, 11.7 and 11.9 years. The error scores also showed little change as a result of drug ingestion, the averages in terms of mental age being 9.7 years (no marihuana), 9.9 years (2 cc.) and 10.2 years (5 cc.), and what change occurred was in a positive direction, that is, there was a very slight improvement in the subject's performance when he was under the influence of marihuana.

Kohs Block Design. This test correlates more highly with abstract intelligence than do any of the other performance tests. Here the drug had a definitely deleterious effect when it was administered in large amounts. The average score was 17.6 when the subjects were not under the influence of marihuana and 14.8 after they had ingested the drug; that is, under 5 cc. of marihuana there was a 16 per cent loss in score as compared with undrugged results.

In general it appears that those functions most closely associated with higher intellectual processes are more impaired by the drug than are the simpler functions.

Memory Tests

Rote Memory. As measured by the ability to repeat digits forward there were no changes in rote memory as a result of drug ingestion, the average scores under no drug, 2 cc. of marihuana, and 5 cc. of marihuana being in each case 7.1.

Digits Reversed. Although the giving of digits in reverse order is always grouped with memory tests, this task actually requires something over and above mere recall. It demands a mental control not necessary in tests dependent purely upon rote memory. Although simple rote memory, as measured by the ability to repeat digits forward, was not affected by the ingestion of marihuana, the repetition of digits reversed was affected adversely. In the undrugged state the average for the group was 5.4, with 2 cc. the average was 5.0, and with 5 cc. it was 4.8. The impairment was comparatively small but it seems to have been related to the amount of drug taken.

Object Memory. The average scores under no drug, 2 cc. of marihuana, and 5 cc. of marihuana were respectively 6.2, 5.6, and 5.9; that is, there was a loss of about 9 per cent in the subject's ability to recall objects which had been exposed to his vision for three seconds when he took the test under the influence of 2 cc. of marihuana, while after the ingestion of 5 cc. the impairment was less, being only about 5 per cent. This seemingly contradictory result is probably due to the fact that by the time the subjects took the test under the influence of 5 cc. most of them had already had it two times previously. The loss in terms of absolute number of remembered articles was slight.

Visual Memory. In this test as in the case of digits reversed something over and above simple memory function is involved. A capacity for analysis and synthesis which correlates well with intelligence is required for the successful execution of this task, and it is this function which is adversely affected by the ingestion of marihuana. The average scores were 10.3 (no drug), 9.7 (2 cc.) and 7.8 (5 cc.); that is, after the ingestion of 2 cc. of marihuana there was a 6 per cent drop in score, while under 5 cc. there was a 24 per cent drop.

In general one may conclude that simple memory functions are not affected by the administration of marihuana while the more complex memory functions are affected adversely, the extent of the impairment being related to the amount of drug taken.

Throughout the examination of subjects on individual tests, the same difference was observed in intensity of the effect upon user and non-user as was noted in group tests.

Experiments with Marihuana Cigarettes

In addition to the tests made to determine the effect of the ingestion of marihuana on various intellectual functions, several experiments were tried with marihuana cigarettes. The tests used in this part of the study were the Bellevue Adult Intelligence Test; the Woody McCall Mixed Fundamentals Test, Form I, which consists of thirty-five examples requiring addition, subtraction, multiplication or division; a cancellation test in which the subject is required to cross out a specific number (in this instance the number 8) wherever it appears on a sheet covered with rows of numbers; the Kohs Block Design Test; and the tests for rote, object, and visual memory.

The subjects took the test series and individual tests twice, once without the drug and once after having smoked marihuana cigarettes. They were not given a specific number of cigarettes but were told to smoke until they felt "high." The number of cigarettes smoked to produce this effect ranged from two to seven.

The Mixed Fundamentals and Cancellation tests were given as group tests and were repeated at half-hour intervals for two and a half hours. In the series given when the subjects were "high," the first test was taken as soon as the cigarettes had been smoked. Time limit on each test was one and a half minutes.

The Bellevue Adult, Kohs, and memory tests were given as individual tests and were administered only twice, once before the subject had smoked marihuana cigarettes and once after he had become "high" from smoking them. If during the course of the examination he wanted another cigarette or the examiner had reason to suspect that he was no longer under the influence of the drug, more cigarettes were smoked. The number of cigarettes used during a three-hour testing period ranged from six to twelve.

In the cancellation, Kohs, and memory tests the subjects were so divided that half took the tests for the first time before they had smoked and half after they had smoked. In the Woody McCall Mixed Fundamentals Test more non-users had their first tests before they had smoked. The Bellevue Adult Intelligence Test was always given first without the drug during the two or three days immediately following the subject's admission. Four weeks later the test was repeated on 10 subjects while they were under the influence of marihuana cigarettes.

Bellevue Adult Intelligence Test

Ten subjects, 5 users and 5 non-users, repeated this test under the influence of marihuana. The results are shown in Table 27.

Table 27

Effect of marihuana cigarettes on I.Q. of ten subjects as measured by the Bellevue Adult Intelligence Test

Dose	Verbal I.Q. Average	Verbal I.Q. Range	Performance I.Q. Average	Performance I.Q. Range	Total I.Q. Average	Total I.Q. Range
Without Cigarettes ..	100.7	88-118	102.3	81-129	101.6	89-124
With Cigarettes	101.8	90-119	106.5	91-135	104.4	94-126

Since the test taken when the subject was "high" was always his second experience with it, some allowance must be made for practice effect. Without drug the average I.Q. of these subjects was 101.6, while after they had smoked cigarettes it was 104.4. This increase of only 2.8 points is smaller than one would probably get with repetition occurring after such a short time interval. It may be concluded, therefore, that smoking marihuana cigarettes has some negative effect on intellectual functioning, in that the subject benefits less from previous experiences than he would if he had not smoked.

Woody McCall Mixed Fundamentals Test, Form I

This test was given to 24 subjects, 10 users and 14 non-users. From the results which are shown in Table 28 it may be concluded that when the subject was "high" after smoking marihuana cigarettes there was a slowing up in his ability to do simple arithmetical calculations. This lag occurred within the first half-hour after smoking and continued for at least an hour. The deleterious effect was not such as to cause an actual loss in ability but the increments resulting from repeated practice were never as great in the drugged as in the undrugged state. Thus, the initial increment was 10 per cent in the test given before smoking and only 4 per cent in the one administered after the subject had become "high." The final increment at the end of two and a half hours was 20 per cent without drug, 13 per cent with drug.

Table 28

Effect of marihuana cigarettes on the ability to use acquired knowledge as measured by the Woody McCall Mixed Fundamentals Test on twenty-four subjects

Time after smoking (in hours)	Before smoking		After smoking	
	Average score*	Increase over initial score (in per cent)	Average score*	Increase over initial score (in per cent)
0	15.0	—	15.9	—
½	16.5	10	16.6	4
1	16.8	12	17.2	8
1½	16.8	12	17.9	13
2	17.9	19	18.8	18
2½	18.0	20	17.8	12

*Score = number of right answers.

This test measures the subject's ability to use acquired knowledge. Under the influence of marihuana cigarettes the capacity for using such an acquired skill is not lost but is slowed down. The adverse effect of smoking marihuana in cigarette form occurs almost immediately in contrast to the delayed action of the pills.

Cancelling 8's

Sixteen subjects, 8 users and 8 non-users, took this test, the results of which are shown in Table 29. As a result of smoking marihuana cigarettes the subject worked a little slower in his execution of a routine task than he did when he had not smoked. The increment over the initial score in the test score made a half-hour after he be-

TABLE 29

Effect of marihuana cigarettes on the ability to carry out a routine task as measured by the cancelling of 8's by sixteen subjects

Time after smoking (in hours)	Before smoking		After smoking	
	Average score*	Increase over initial score (in per cent)	Average score*	Increase over initial score (in per cent)
0	50.0	—	48.4	—
½	54.7	9	51.6	7
1	55.3	11	49.7	3
1½	57.2	14	56.2	16
2	54.0	8	51.6	7
2½	57.2	14	58.1	20

*Score = number of right answers—number of wrong answers.

came "high" was only 7 per cent as against an increment of 9 per cent when the cigarettes had not been smoked. His performance was slowed up for one hour after smoking and possibly longer.

KOHS BLOCK DESIGN TEST

This test, which measures performance ability, was given to a total of 9 subjects, 6 users and 3 non-users. The average score without the drug was 18.5, and after cigarettes have been smoked 14.7. This difference in score of 3.8 points indicates a loss in efficiency of 21 per cent.

MEMORY TESTS

Rote Memory. Thirteen users and 9 non-users took this test. Neither in repeating digits forward nor in giving them in reverse did the subjects show any disadvantageous effects from the use of marihuana cigarettes, the average scores before and after smoking being 6.9 and 7.1 respectively for the digits forward test and 5.2 and 5.1 for the digits reversed test. The only explanation for this deviation from the results obtained when marihuana was taken in pill form is the inability to control the dosage when marihuana is given in cigarette form.

Object Memory. Thirteen subjects took this test. Object memory was not impaired by the smoking of marihuana, the average scores being 6.8 before the cigarettes were smoked and 7.1 when the subjects were "high."

Visual Memory. There was an .8 point loss (from 10.5 to 9.7) in the average score of the 20 subjects, 11 users and 9 non-users, who took this test. This represents an impairment of about 8 per cent.

Effect of Marihuana Cigarettes on Users and Non-Users

The difference in intensity of effect of marihuana cigarettes on the user and on the non-user was not the same as the difference in the effect of the marihuana concentrate on these two groups. The user was usually more affected by smoking marihuana than was the non-user, probably because the non-user did not smoke as much or as intensely as the user and was not as much under the influence of the drug.

Effects on Women

Five women were used in this experiment, 1 marihuana user and 4 non-users. The group as a whole was of average intelligence, with an I.Q. of 101.3, range 85 to 115, on Bellevue Adult Intelligence Test. Verbal I.Q. was 101.0, range 89 to 116; performance I.Q. 101.5, range 83 to 117. Average age for the group was 30.3 years, range 28 to 34.

The tests used and the procedure employed were the same for the women as for the men with the following exceptions: (1) the Army Alpha test was given every hour instead of every half-hour; (2) no form board tests were given; (3) no group tests with cigarettes were given.

Test results for the female subjects were not entirely like those obtained for the men. In the case of the woman, intellectual impairment, as measured by Army Alpha total scores, was more severe and lasting under 2 cc. of marihuana than it was under 3 to 5 cc. This was also true of learning ability as measured by Pyle's Digit Symbol test. The ability to carry out a routine task showed impairment only when tested under the influence of 3 to 5 cc. of the drug. The ingestion of the drug in either dosage brought about an improvement in rote memory (digits forward), while in the digits reversed test there was an impairment under 2 cc. and no change under 5 cc. Object memory remained unchanged when the subject had had 2 cc. of marihuana, and was slightly impaired with 3 to 5 cc. and cigarettes. There was a drop in score for visual memory (Army Designs Test) under both 2 cc. and 5 cc. of the drug. Kohs Block Design Test (a performance test which requires integrative functioning at higher intellectual levels) was given only twice, once without the drug and once with 5 cc. There was a loss in efficiency on this test when taken under marihuana which was comparable to that reported for the men.

It should be noted that the performance of the female subjects showed great variability. This variability may have been due either to the small number of subjects employed, or to their special selection, or both, and the findings can only be considered suggestive of possible trends. The fact that in some tests the subjects were more adversely affected by 2 cc. of marihuana than by larger doses is probably due to the fact that the 2 cc. dose was always administered before the larger dosage, and possibly also to the seemingly greater suggestibility of this particular group of women.

Conclusions

1. Marihuana taken either in pill or in cigarette form has a transitory adverse effect on mental functioning.

2. The extent of intellectual impairment, the time of its onset, and its duration are all related to the amount of drug taken. Small doses cause only slight falling off in mental ability while larger doses result in greater impairment. The deleterious effect is measurable earlier with large doses than with small ones, and the impairment continues for a greater length of time with large doses than with small ones.

3. The degree of intellectual impairment resulting from the presence of marihuana in the system varies with the function tested. The more complex functions are more severely affected than the simpler ones.

4. In general, non-users experience greater intellectual impairment for longer periods of time than the users do. This suggests the possibility of an habituation factor.

5. The falling off in ability which occurs when an individual has taken marihuana is due to a loss in both speed and accuracy.

6. Indulgence in marihuana does not appear to result in mental deterioration.

EMOTIONAL REACTIONS AND GENERAL PERSONALITY STRUCTURE

FLORENCE HALPERN, M.A.

The purpose of this part of the study was twofold: to discover (1) what effect marihuana has on the emotional reactivity of the person taking it; and (2) what differences in emotional reaction and general personality structure exist between the marihuana user and non-user.

Tests

Two types of tests are available for studying personality. These are the paper-pencil tests and the projective tests. Projective techniques which reveal the subject's personality through his treatment of the test material are generally more valid and more revealing than the paper-pencil tests which require the underlining of words or the answering of "Yes" or "No" to a list of questions. This is true of all subjects but seemed to apply more particularly to those used in this study. Such tests as the Psychosomatic Inventory and the Bell Adjustment Test were tried out in the initial stages of the investigation but were soon discontinued as the subjects gave continued evidence of a desire to ingratiate themselves with, or to make a showing for, the examiner. Questions whose intent was obvious were almost invariably answered as the subject thought the examiner wanted them to be or as he thought would look best on his record. For this reason most of the tests employed were those whose purposes were less easily interpreted by the subjects.

RORSCHACH TEST

One of the primary tests employed for examining the personality of the subjects was the Rorschach Test. It consists of ten standardized ink blots printed on 7 by 9½ inch white cards. Some of the blots are black, some red and black, and some multicolored. The cards are presented to the subject one at a time and he states what they look like to him, what he sees. The manner in which the subject interprets the plates gives an indication of his formal approach to various types of situations. The extent and directions of the subject's affective reactions, his drive, his ability to make good social adjustment and his emotional stability are some of the personality traits which can be determined on the basis of this test.

Goodenough Test (Drawing of a Man)

This test was standardized originally as an intelligence test for children, but clinical use has demonstrated its value as an instrument for personality diagnosis. The subject is given a sheet of paper 8½ by 11 inches and asked to draw the figure of a man. In his drawing he unconsciously portrays his own body image so that the picture by its emphasis and omissions betrays which body parts are important or unimportant to him—how he sees himself. Although results from this type of interpretation have not, to our knowledge, been standardized, they may nevertheless be used for comparing the marihuana user and non-user in terms of their attitudes toward their body images and for noting the differences in these concepts before and after the administration of marihuana.

Level of Aspiration Test

The purpose of a Level of Aspiration Test is to ascertain the relationship between the goal a person sets for himself and the level of his performance. Roughly, there are three possible reactions: (1) the individual, in an attempt to protect his ego, sets himself so low a goal that he must inevitably reach or surpass it; (2) he exposes his ego to failure by overevaluating his ability and sets a goal which he cannot possibly reach or surpass; or (3) he sets a goal commensurate with his ability.

The test devised for this experiment is a very simple one. The subject is required to place sixteen colored cubes in a box, red side up. Before beginning he is asked to estimate how long it will take to complete the task. He is then given the signal to proceed and at the end of the trial is told how much time was actually consumed. On the basis of this result, the subject is again asked to state how much time he thinks he will need to fulfill the task and again at its completion is told how long it actually took him. The subject's estimate given before he had any actual experience with the test is disregarded. From the nine subsequent trials, averages of the subject's estimate (the goal he set for himself) and of his actual performance times are calculated. The difference between these two averages gives a measure of his level of aspiration.

Frustration Test

When a person is prevented from finishing a task correctly, thus being left with an incomplete gestalt, he has definite feelings of frustration. His reactions to such feelings will vary depending upon his general manner of emotional response. In this investigation, the method used to frustrate the subjects was to present them with a series of relatively simple mazes (Wechsler Self-Administering Mazes), the third or fourth one being so blocked off that no exit is possible. The subject is highly praised for his performance on the first two or three and, when he becomes involved in the closed one, is aggravated by the comments of the examiner concerning the success of some of the other men with this identical maze. After fifteen seconds of futile attempts to get out the subject is told that his time is up. Immediately after this he is given the Level of Aspiration Test, the assumption being that frustration might affect this level in some way.

Binet Lines

Suggestibility is a specific rather than a general trait and can therefore be interpreted only with reference to the situation in which it is tested. For example, a man may be very responsive to the suggestions of his attractive secretary but negativistic to those of his business rival.

Binet's Suggestibility Test, which consists of twelve rectangular pieces of cardboard on which are drawn lines of varying length, was used in this investigation. The length of the first five lines increases by specific amounts; the sixth line does not increase but is identical with the fifth; the seventh line again is longer; the eighth is its equivalent; and so on. The assumption is that the progressive increase of the first five lines will influence the suggestible person and he will continue to increase the lines for some time before he becomes aware of the fact that they are no longer consistently lengthening.

The following directions are given: "I want to see how well you can estimate length. I am going to show you some cards, each with a line drawn on it. Some of the lines are long and some are short. I'll show you each card for just two seconds and when I take it away you must draw the line. Try to make it exactly the length of the line on the card." The subject is given a sheet of paper which has a vertical line drawn about half an inch in from the left-hand edge of the paper. Numbers, placed about half an inch apart, appear inside this margin, beginning at the top with number 1 and going through number 12. The subject is told to begin his line opposite the number and right up against the vertical-line margin. As soon as he has drawn his line it is covered with the card and the next card is presented.

Results are scored in accordance with Binet's method. The average amount of increase (measured in sixteenths of an inch) for the even lines which actually should not increase is divided by the average increase in the odd lines which should increase, and the quotient is multiplied by 100.

Wechsler Vocational Interest Blank

The Wechsler Vocational Interest Blank consists of a list of forty jobs or vocations, each followed by the letter "L" or "D." These vocations may be classed as professional, artistic, industrial, or manual. The subject is told that for the moment he is to assume that each job pays the same amount and that he has the training and ability to do any of them. The only thing to influence his choice of a job is his own inclination, that is, whether or not that type of work appeals to him. If it does he is told to encircle the "L," but if it does not he is to encircle the "D." The choice of certain constellations of jobs, such as painting, teaching, and working in a florist shop, indicates a general feminine trend, while preference for others gives evidence of strongly masculine inclinations. Again, the selection of many positions may be taken to indicate an active, outgoing nature, while a small number of likes reflects a less active, more critical attitude.

Loofbourrow Personal Index: Test I

This test is given to adolescent boys to measure their proneness to delinquency. In this study it was employed as a measure of self-confidence. It consists of one hundred words of which thirty are nonexistent, that is, words which look like unusual but real words but which are actually not part of the English language. If at any time, drugged or undrugged, a subject indicates familiarity with a significantly larger number of words than on another occasion, the assumption is that the increase in vocabulary corresponds to a rise in the subject's estimate of his own ability and mental capacity.

Wechsler Free Association Test

This test consists of a list of forty-five words chosen for their obvious value in personality study. The examiner reads the words one at a time to the subject and records his responses and his reaction time in fifths of a second. Reaction times and average deviation are computed for each subject, and those words for which the reaction time is delayed, that is, words which fall beyond the limits of the average deviation, are considered disturbing stimuli.

Pressey X-O Test

There are four parts to this test, each one consisting of twenty-five lines of five words each. In Test I the subject is asked to cross out every word whose meaning is unpleasant to him and to encircle the one word in each row whose meaning is the most unpleasant. In Test II each row of words is preceded by a word in large print and the subject is instructed to cross out every word in the row which is connected in his mind with the word in large letters at the beginning of the row. At the end of this test the subject encircles the one word in each row which he most closely associates with the word in large letters. Test III requires the subject to cross out every word he thinks has a bad meaning and then to encircle the one thing in each row he thinks is worst. Test IV follows the same procedure, only here the subject crosses out everything he has ever worried about and encircles the one thing in each row he has worried about most. Norms have been established on college students, giving the average number of words crossed out and the modal word to be encircled.

Downey Will-Temperament Test: Test I

This test consists of a series of paired personality traits such as sociable or unsociable, clumsy or graceful. The subject is asked to underscore the trait of each pair which he thinks describes him more accurately. The test is not intended as a self-rating personality index, and therefore there are no norms for responses of this nature. It was used in this study solely to determine if the ingestion of marihuana produces changes in the individual's self-evaluation as indicated by a comparison of the traits he thinks apply to him when he is in his normal condition and when he is under the influence of the drug.

Thematic Apperception Test

This test employs a series of pictures which are handed to the subject one at a time with the following directions: "This is a test of creative imagination. I am going to show you some pictures. Around each picture I want you to compose a story. Outline the incidents which have led up to the situation shown in the picture; describe what is occurring at the moment—the feelings and thoughts of the characters; and tell what the outcome will be. Speak your thoughts aloud as they come to your mind. I want you to use your imagination to the limit." Productions are recorded verbatim. Scoring takes into account the needs of the subject as revealed in his stories and the environmental forces acting upon him.

Procedure

All the tests dealing with emotional reactions were given as individual tests. Although they are not as subject to practice effect as the Intelligence tests, practice does alter the results somewhat. For this reason every possible effort was made to give examinations during drugged and undrugged periods as far apart in time as possible and to divide the groups so that half the subjects took the initial examination while under the influence of marihuana and the other half before the administration of the drug.

Rorschach Test

This test was given once without marihuana and once under maximum dosage (3 cc. to 6 cc.) or with cigarettes, the number of cigarettes smoked being optional with the subject. Four subjects took the test three times, once without the drug, once with the drug in pill form, and once with cigarettes, but it was found impracticable to give the test more than twice in four weeks both because of the time it consumed and because of the subjects' growing boredom with it. In all, 45 subjects, 27 users and 18 non-users, took this test.

Goodenough, Level of Aspiration, Binet Lines, and Vocational Interest Tests, Downey Test I

These tests were given to all subjects at least twice and some subjects took them as often as four times, that is, without the drug, under 2 cc., under 5 cc., and after smoking marihuana cigarettes. The number of times a subject was tested was determined primarily by the amount of time available. Twenty-seven users and 18 non-users took the Goodenough, Level of Aspiration and Vocational Interest Tests; 25 users and 17 non-users the Binet Lines; and 14 users and 8 non-users the Downey Will-Temperament Test.

Frustration, Free Association, and Pressey X-O Tests, and Loofbourrow Test I

These tests were added later in the testing program and were therefore given to a limited number of subjects. They were administered twice, once without marihuana and once either with cigarettes or with large oral doses (3 cc. to 5 cc.)

Thematic Apperception Test

In an effort to conserve time, the administration of this test was not in accordance with the directions. Instead of relating the story to the examiner, the subject sat in a room by himself and recited his tale into the dictaphone. In addition to the time saved, this had the advantage of sparing the subject considerable embarrassment, since most of the men were very self-conscious about telling these stories when anyone was present. The disadvantage of this procedure lay in the examiner's inability to persuade the subject to give a fuller story. The test was given to each subject twice, once with and once without cigarettes. Only the following pictures were used: 3, 4, 5, M-11, M-12, M-13, M-15, M-18, M-19, M-20, F-14, and F-19. Although the results showed promise of interesting findings, the administration of the test was limited to only 9 subjects because so many mechanical difficulties were involved.

Findings

Rorschach Test

Table 30 gives the Rorschach findings for 45 subjects both in the undrugged and drugged states. The measurable changes on the test which occurred during the period of drug intoxication were few and not far-reaching. They may be considered indications of tendencies rather than of significant alterations of the personality.

TABLE 30

Effect of marihuana on personality structure as shown on the Rorschach Test

	45 subjects		27 users		18 non-users	
	Without Marihuana	With Marihuana	Without Marihuana	With Marihuana	Without Marihuana	With Marihuana
Average number of responses	20.0	23.3	19.4	21.5	20.8	26.2
Type of response (per cent of total)						
Whole	40	36	36	34	46	39
Detail	43	42	47	43	38	40
Rare detail	17	21	17	22	16	21
Form	57	56	62	59	50	52
Form +	92	86	92	90	93	82
Ms	11	10	9	9	13	10
C	10	9	9	8	11	10
Chiaroscuro	14	15	11	14	17	16
FM + m	12	12	11	11	14	13
A	36 }54	35 }51	37 }58	36 }55	35 }48	34 }48
Ad	18	16	21	19	13	14
H	13	13	11	11	14	14
Hd	8	9	8	10	7	8
P	27	20	29	20	25	19
M:C	2.3:1.6	2.9:2.1				

When the subjects were under the influence of marihuana (either 3-6 cc. or cigarettes, the number of cigarettes being at the discretion of the smoker) there was a slightly freer flow of associations than there was when they were in the undrugged state, an increased productivity which coincided with the impressions obtained from general observation of the subjects when they were "high." Without drug the average number of interpretations made was 20.0, with drug 23.3. This increased number of responses was due primarily to the subject's greater awareness of small, extraneous details which in his undrugged state he overlooked. Thus, while 17 per cent of the subjects' answers were small or rare detail responses when no marihuana had been administered, with marihuana this increased to 21 per cent. Coincidental with his increased absorption in the irrelevant there was a slight decrease in the subject's drive to organize and synthesize. Whereas without drug 40 per cent of the responses involved the entire blot, with drug this was true of only 36 per cent of the interpretations. Under the influence of marihuana there was a mild tendency for the subject to become preoccupied with minutiae rather than to concern himself with the larger, more important aspects of a situation, and this implies some falling off in meaningful constructive behavior.

When the subject had taken marihuana there was some decrease in the objectivity with which he sized up situations. This was indicated by the fact that without drug 92 per cent of his interpretations were good form, that is, they corresponded to the form of the blot, while with drug this percentage fell to 86 per cent. The drug had an adverse effect on the individual's critical faculty and he was more prone to jump to erroneous conclusions than he was when he was in the undrugged state.

The only other change that occurred on the Rorschach test after the ingestion of marihuana was the decrease in the subject's ability to think in line with the group. This showed itself in the decreased number of popular interpretations made, the drop being from 27 per cent without drug to 20 per cent with drug. In other words, during the period of drug intoxication an individual is somewhat less likely to see the obvious and the commonplace than he is in his normal state.

As important, or possibly even more important, than the changes which occurred on the Rorschach after ingestion or smoking of marihuana, is the fact that some of the most basic personality attributes remained unchanged. Thus it appeared that 33 per cent of the subjects in the undrugged state were what is described as introversive, that is, they were individuals who tend to withdraw somewhat from the world about them and depend primarily on their own inner resources for emotional stimulation; 20 per cent were extraversive, depending mainly on their environment for affective satisfaction; 20 per cent were ambivert showing equal potentialities in both directions; and 27 per cent were emotionally constricted to the point where they gave little or no evidence of emotional response of any type. With drug 36 per cent were introversive, 22 per cent were extraversive, 20 per cent were ambivert, and 22 per cent were constricted. Marihuana ingestion or smoking served to dilate the emotional life of only 2 of the subjects and shifted the type of 1. In all 3 cases the change was actually a very slight one. The fact that the emotional trends remain essentially unchanged under the influence of marihuana was further revealed by the fact that the ratio for evaluating the individual's emotional type, that is, the ratio of movement to color, remained roughly the same before and after he had taken the drug, being 2.3:1.6 when he was in the undrugged state and 2.9:2.1 when he was in the drugged phase.

Although the quantitative changes occurring with marihuana ingestion or smoking were not large, there was a qualitative difference in the protocols obtained from the subjects in the undrugged and drugged stages. Not only was there a slight increase in the actual number of interpretations made, but the amount of talking and extraneous comment increased. The subject played around with his answers and often repeated them. He seemed anxious to get his every thought clearly across to his audience. More than this, he was much freer in the type of interpretation he allowed himself. For example, one interpretation on Card II read: "Two dogs. Now wait a minute. I don't want to jump to conclusions but it looks as if the dogs were having intercourse and there was a rupture." This response was not repeated when the subject was retested in the undrugged state. Nor was this individual unique in showing this qualitative difference. The disinhibition and lessening of restraint which was a definitely observable effect of the drug was also reflected in the assured explanations and lengthy tirades which the subject offered on topics which in his undrugged state he would undoubtedly feel were beyond him. Thus one subject interpreted Card X as "old bark of trees, roots dried up. It's thousands of years old; it takes thousands of years to do that. I got to tell you that. I got to cover for you. You wouldn't know about a thousand years ago. I'm smart now." In some instances the "cockiness" induced by his drugged condition produced an entirely new attitude in the subject. Instead of the customary deferential, almost ingratiating approach there was now a confident "know-it-all" manner.

The effects of marihuana ingestion on user and non-user were essentially the same, as indicated by the findings in Table 30, except that on the whole the alterations which did occur were more marked for the non-user than for the user. Thus, for example, while the average number of responses given by the user increased only 11 per cent, those of the non-user rose 26 per cent. Again, the user when drugged gave only 6 per cent fewer whole answers as against a decrease of 15 per cent in the whole responses of the non-user in the drugged state. The user showed a 29 per cent increase in small detail interpretations, the non-user 31 per cent. There was only a 2 per cent drop in good form interpretation by the user as against a 12 per cent drop for the non-user. Only in the loss of popular interpretations did the user exceed the non-user, his falling off being as great as 31 per cent as compared with 24 per cent for the non-user. While the number of subjects in both groups was too small to allow of definite statements, the trend seemed to indicate that the ingestion or smoking of marihuana has a greater adverse or disorganizing effect on the neophyte than on the experienced smoker, again, as was the case in the study of mental functioning, suggesting the possibility of psychological habituation.

When the protocols obtained from these marihuana users in their undrugged state are compared with those of the non-users or with the norms postulated for average adults of this age level, certain deviating personality traits in these users may be noted. The most striking deviation is the small percentage of users who showed an extraversive personality. Only 15 per cent of the marihuana users used in this study responded primarily to emotional stimuli in the world about them as compared with 28 per cent of the non-users. While no definite figures are given in the literature for the degree of extraversion in the general population, it seems definitely more than 15 per cent. Altogether the personality types among the non-users show a much more even distribution than those among the users as seen in Table 31. Judging by the personality types the majority of marihuana users lack social ease and adroitness and are likely to find it difficult to make good outgoing social contacts.

TABLE 31

Personality types of user and non-user subjects as shown on the Rorschach Test

Personality Types	Users	Non-Users
Extraversive	15%	28%
Introversive	37%	28%
Ambivert	19%	28%
Constricted	30%	17%

Sixty-two per cent of the marihuana users' interpretations were determined by the form or outline of the blot. Such responses require an objective critical attitude unmodified by emotional factors. However, when this attitude is maintained to the point where more than 50 per cent of the answers are of this nature the individual has a constricted affective life, the degree of constriction being in proportion to the increase in form interpretations. Thus, as was previously noted, there was more than average emotional inhibition evident among the marihuana users studied in this experiment. Since emotional inhibition frequently causes intellectual constriction, it is not surprising to find that the stereotypy in these records was slightly above expectancy, as indicated by the fact that 59 per cent of the responses were animal or animal detail interpretations as compared with a norm of from 25 to 50 per cent.

Finally the marihuana users (as well as the non-users in this experiment) showed a depressive outlook in that more of their responses were determined by the gray and black colors than by the vivid colors. In interpreting this fact it must be borne in mind that the subjects were all prisoners and their depressive attitude may have been a reflection of their present situation rather than of a basic trait.

Goodenough Test (Drawing of a Man)

This test is helpful in studying each individual both in the drugged and undrugged state, but group results are not meaningful (except for one finding given below) because of a lack of similarity both in the drawings obtained in the undrugged state and in the direction of change which occurred after drug ingestion or smoking. However, certain qualitative findings proved interesting and are therefore reported here. In a number of cases the identical drawing was produced in the undrugged, 2 cc., 5 cc., and cigarette state, but the size of the figure increased consistently with the amount of marihuana taken. This increase in size may have been a reflection of a physical sensation induced by the drug, may have been due to a tendency to macrographia which was noted in the writing of some subjects, or may have been the psychological representation of increased feelings of confidence and security.

With marihuana there was an increase in the percentage of subjects who remembered to give their man ears. This again may have been due to a heightened awareness of ears because of physical or auditory sensations or might denote a greater receptivity to what others have to say.

In some cases the amount of time consumed in execution of the drawings was considerably greater when the subject was "high." This additional time was rarely used for elaborating the picture but was caused by the subject's altered mood. In many instances the laughter and joking in which he indulged kept him from completing the job with dispatch. In other cases depression or nausea slowed him up. Although aware of the details which should be included, the subject was often satisfied to indicate such items by a single line or dash rather than discipline himself to the point where he could make a careful picture. In some of these cases the drawing had attributes which resemble the findings sometimes seen in productions of individuals in a manic mood.

When a person is given a sheet of paper and is asked to draw a man on it, the paper and the figure he draws become the situation he must manipulate. If the figure is well centered so that the finished product gives a balanced composition, the subject has handled the circumstance in adequate fashion. The one consistent finding for this test was the fact that the subject's ability to handle situations was not improved by drug ingestion or smoking. In the case of both user and non-user the percentage of balanced compositions produced in the various drug states did not change from the results obtained in the undrugged condition. It is, however, interesting to note that 59 per cent of the marihuana users made "unbalanced" drawings in the undrugged state as compared with only 29 per cent of the non-users. It may be inferred from this that fewer users than non-users are inclined to come out into the center of the scene. This carries with it implications of poor adjustment and insecurity.

Level of Aspiration Test

In the undrugged state the majority of the subjects manifested reactions which are usual in the experience of other experiments, namely, the tendency to place their estimate just a little above their actual performance. This was demonstrated by the fact that while the average performance time needed for carrying out a set task (putting sixteen blocks in a box, red side up) was 23.6 seconds, the subjects' average estimate for accomplishing this was 21.9 seconds. As their performance improved with practice, the subjects tended to allow themselves less time for the job. Such statements as, "I should do better this time," or, "I'll take a chance," were not infrequent. Some subjects wanted to know the best score ever made, and worked energetically to attain it.

With 2 cc. of marihuana there was a slight increase in the average estimated time for the entire group although there was no concomitant increase in performance time. Under this dosage the estimated time was 23.1 seconds, performance time 23.4 seconds. Although the subject actually took no longer to do the job, he thought he would work more slowly and in predicting his achievement gave himself more time. His attitude during the test was a much easier, more happy-go-lucky one. He occasionally stopped in the middle of the experiment to discuss something with the examiner or call out to someone passing in the hall. There thus appeared to be a small loss in drive which, though not revealed by significant statistical differences, was indicated by the numerical trend and by the subject's attitude toward the test.

After the ingestion of 5 cc. of marihuana the average estimated time was 23.2 seconds and the performance time 24.4 seconds. Here the relationship between estimated and performance time was similar to that found in the undrugged phase, that is, there was a 1.2-second gap between them. During this drug phase the subjects seemed less relaxed than they were under 2 cc., and their main interest seemed to be to get back to bed and be left undisturbed.

Under the influence of marihuana cigarettes the trend was similar to that found with 2 cc., the difference between the estimated time and the performance time being only .3 seconds. As with 2 cc., the subject's behavior was generally happy and relaxed.

When the group was divided into users and non-users the trend was the same for both.

TABLE 32

Average time estimated and taken for Level of Aspiration Test

Dose	Average time (in seconds)								
	Users and non-users			Users			Non-users		
	Est.	Perf.	Diff.	Est.	Perf.	Diff.	Est.	Perf.	Diff.
0 cc.	21.9	23.6	1.7	22.1	23.5	1.4	21.8	23.6	1.8
2 cc.	23.1	23.4	.3	23.7	23.7	0.0	22.6	23.1	.5
5 cc.	23.2	24.4	1.2	23.7	25.0	1.3	22.7	23.8	1.1
Cigs.	24.1	24.4	.3	24.1	24.7	.6	24.1	24.1	0.0

On the whole it appears that small doses of marihuana and of marihuana cigarettes tend to lower the individual level of aspiration, that is, there is a slight lessening in the subject's drive and his will to achieve. Larger doses (5 cc.) do not produce this effect.

Frustration Test

The results of the frustration experiment indicated no statistically significant differences between the subject's reactions before and after he had taken marihuana. Again, after the ingestion of marihuana there was a slight trend toward lowering the level of aspiration (Table 33), but the over-all change was not startling when compared with results on the Level of Aspiration Test when no frustrating experience was introduced.

Table 33

Average time estimated and taken for Frustration Test

Dose	Average time (in seconds)								
	Users and non-users			Users			Non-users		
	Est.	Perf.	Diff.	Est.	Perf.	Diff.	Est.	Perf.	Diff.
0 cc.	21.4	22.6	1.2	21.5	22.7	1.2	21.3	22.4	1.1
5 cc.	23.6	23.1	0.5	24.5	23.2	1.3	22.7	23.0	0.3
Cigs.	22.6	22.6	0.0	23.1	23.1	0.0	22.0	22.0	0.0

Binet Lines

Binet's interpretation of this test was based upon the principle that suggestible individuals, once embarked on a particular form of activity (in this instance, drawing lines of increasing length), are more prone to continue this activity when the stimulus is altered than are less suggestible people. Judging by the results as given in Table 34, small doses of marihuana (2 cc. and cigarettes) induced this type of perseverative behavior in the users but not in the non-users. In other words, the marihuana user when under the influence of the drug tended to continue an activity he had started without being too discriminatory or controlled about it. The non-user, on the other hand, showed a curtailment in activity and responsiveness. One possible explanation of this difference in effect on user and non-user appears to lie in the fact that the drug made the user more relaxed and easy-going and less controlled in motor activity than he was in his undrugged state, while the non-user was often more tense and disturbed. As was so often the case in the personality tests, the effect on the user of large doses of the drug (5 cc.) was contrary to that of the small ones, probably because in many cases he was made physically uncomfortable and intellectually disorganized.

TABLE 34

Average scores on the Binet Lines Test

Dose	Users	Non-Users
0 cc.	90.2	99.2
2 cc.	105.9	60.9
5 cc.	81.1	98.7
Cigs.	106.3	87.3

The lack of consistency in the findings seems to suggest that the individual's psychological and physiological "set" toward the drug affects his reaction and behavior. Thus small doses, which the marihuana user anticipates with pleasure, make him more easy-going and therefore probably more suggestible than he would be in his undrugged state, while large doses have a contrary effect. The non-user, on the other hand, appears to be less suggestible as a result of drug ingestion than he ordinarily is.

WECHSLER VOCATIONAL INTEREST BLANK

The average number of positions chosen by the subjects when they were in the undrugged state was 13.2. With 2 cc. of marihuana the average was 12.9; with 5 cc., 12.7; and with cigarettes, 11.8. There was a very slight but not statistically significant trend toward a decrease in job interest. However, the absence of any appreciable change in the number of positions liked after the ingestion or smoking of marihuana indicates that no real withdrawal is implied.

Analysis of the type of position chosen shows that under the influence of marihuana there was no swing to the more feminine occupations, but in the case of some subjects, especially marihuana users, there was a falling off in the popularity of some jobs which require considerable activity. For example, under the influence of 2 cc. of marihuana or of marihuana cigarettes the jobs of detective, policeman and taxi driver were found among his least desired occupations though they were not in this place when he was in the undrugged state.

The trend was the same for the user and the non-user in both the drugged and undrugged phase. For the user the jobs of aviator, gymnasium teacher, newspaper reporter, sailor and soldier were most frequently chosen; for the non-user aviator, doctor, explorer, forest ranger, newspaper reporter and prize fighter were most popular.

LOOFBOURROW PERSONAL INDEX: TEST I

Before taking marihuana, the user and non-user on an average indicated familiarity with an identical number of words, 65.2. After he had smoked marihuana cigarettes, the user's vocabulary showed a gain of 6 words, the non-user's 5 words. In both cases the subject's confidence in his verbal capacity was enhanced by the use of marihuana.

WECHSLER FREE ASSOCIATION TEST

In the undrugged state the user and the non-user were disturbed by the same stimulus words, namely "lonely," "passionate," "insult," and "sin." The only differences were the disturbance the user showed in response to the words "wish" and "murder" and the delayed reaction of the non-user to the word "pity."

Under the influence of 5 cc. of marihuana or of marihuana cigarettes the user was less disturbed by all these words with the possible exception of "insult," but there was a sharp increase in the agitation aroused by the words "suicide" and "death." It appears that the feeling of well-being produced by the drug tended to alleviate the loneliness, guilt, and frustration which the subject felt, but it was also accompanied by a fear of death. This may be tied up with the anxiety the marihuana user always experiences in regard to the amount of drug he is taking, the always present fear of his "blowing his top," or it may be a reflection of the problems which were most disturbing to him.

The non-user, after taking marihuana, was also less disturbed by the words "lonely," "passionate," and "sin." His reaction to "pity" was also diminished but he, too, was still upset by the word "insult." The new disturbing stimulus words were not those which upset the user but those which were more closely related to his own immediate problems, namely "honest," "money," and "sex." Since the non-user in our group was generally an individual who had been sent to prison because of stealing or a sex offense, it seems it was these problems which the disinhibiting action of the drug brought to the fore.

Pressey X-O Test

This test was taken by only 10 subjects, 5 users and 5 non-users. In general, the smoking of marihuana brought about some increase in the number of words which had an unpleasant meaning to the subject and in the number of things about which he had worried. There was some decrease in the number of things for which the drugged subject thought a person should be blamed. The number of his associations with any one word remained roughly the same in the drugged and undrugged state.

Although less inclined to censure when under the influence of marihuana, the subject was nevertheless more readily disturbed and worried. This undercurrent of irritability and anxiety seemed to be a concomitant of the more obvious feeling of general well-being which is the predominant effect of the drug. Two possible explanations can be given here for this finding: the physiological changes occurring with the smoking of the drug gave the subject a feeling of anxiety, and the disinhibition which occurred at this time released the restraints which had been imposed not only on the happier reactions but on all the repressed unpleasantness as well, and things which the subject had repressed because he wished to forget them now came to the fore. This was noted when at least two of the subjects had "crying jags" when drugged, reproaching themselves for what they had done to their mothers and wives.

Table 35

Average number of words marked in Pressey X-O Test

Tests		Without Marihuana	With Cigarettes
Test I			
(No. of words with unpleasant meaning)			
	Average	48.4	58.2
	Range	26-76	34-106
Test II			
(No. of words associated with the stimulus word)			
	Average	32.5	34.4
	Range	25-48	25-54
Test III			
(No. of things subject thinks are wrong)			
	Average	79.0	64.5
	Range	48-86	27-99
Test IV			
(No. of things subject has worried about)			
	Average	31.3	42.1
	Range	23-41	26-62

Downey Will-Temperament Test: Test I

The changes in the subjects' responses on this test showed a shift in their attitude toward themselves as a result of marihuana ingestion. On the whole, more subjects appeared to think better of themselves when they were "high" than they did in their undrugged state. This is indicated by the fact that there was an increase in the number of individuals who under the influence of 5 cc. of marihuana or of marihuana cigarettes believed themselves to be careful, cautious, ambitious, accurate, industrious, impulsive, enthusiastic, and possessing superior characters. There was also a decrease in the number who considered themselves suggestible or extravagant. The only negative traits which the subject admitted to more frequently when he was "high" than he did in his normal state were suggestibility, poor memory and aggression. The change in attitude in regard to aggression was most striking among the marihuana users, 88 per cent of whom considered themselves aggressive after they had had the drug as compared with only 42 per cent in the undrugged state. This increase in the feeling of aggression was not paralleled by the findings of the other tests nor by the behavior of the subjects when they had taken the drug. Like the increased vocabulary noted on the Loofbourrow it can best be interpreted as an indication of the subject's increased feelings of confidence and self-assurance.

In general the changes which occurred on this test after the subject had had marihuana were not consistent for the user and the non-user or for different amounts of the drug. They merely served to indicate that when the subject was under the influence of marihuana there were shifts in his feelings about himself which reflected a prevailing mood of confidence and self-satisfaction.

Thematic Apperception Test

Without cigarettes the needs most frequently expressed in the subjects' stories were "affiliation," "aggression," "sex," "dominance," "succorance," "self-abasement," and "play." These terms may be defined as follows:* Affiliation: to be sociable, to make friends, to love. Aggression: to fight, to criticize, to blame, to accuse or ridicule maliciously, to injure or kill, sadism. Sex: to seek sex objects, to court, to enjoy intercourse. Dominance: to influence or control

*Directions for Thematic Apperception Test prepared by Robert W. White and R. Nevitt-Sanford, Harvard Psychological Clinic, February 1941.

others, leadership. Succorance: to seek aid, protection or sympathy. Self-abasement: to comply, to surrender, to accept punishment, to apologize, to condone, to atone, to depreciate the ego, masochism. Play: to relax tension and alleviate stress by pleasurable and humorously irresponsible activity, motor, verbal or mental.

In general the frequency with which all needs were expressed fell off after the subjects had smoked marihuana cigarettes. The most striking drops were in the need for self-abasement and aggression where the frequency of occurrence changed from 2.4 to 1.1 for the former, and from 2.7 to 1.7 for the latter. Contrary to the general trend there was an increase in the need for dominance.

When the subjects were not "high" the environmental influences most frequently mentioned in their stories were illness and death and accepting parents. After smoking marihuana the general trend was similar to that noted for the "needs," that is, there was a falling off in the frequency with which the subjects used most of the concepts. There was, however, no diminution in the number of times that illness and death played a part in their tales, the average number being 2.1 before smoking and 2.2 after smoking. Likewise the awareness of restraint and imprisonment remained constant, occurring 1.1 times before smoking and 1.2 after. Contrary to the general trend there was an increased awareness of an accepting love object. This concept appeared in the stories on an average of .8 times before smoking and 1.2 after.

The decrease in the number of times both needs and environmental pressures were expressed in the stories given after the subjects had had cigarettes was not due to a curtailment in the length of the story. The tales were often more wordy in the drugged than in the undrugged state, but their length was frequently due to embellishment and repetition, and there was likely to be less meaningful material. In general the stories obtained from the subjects after smoking indicated that they had less capacity for expressing themselves directly and clearly, and also less concern with self-abasement and aggression. As defined on this test these needs represent a conflict between aggression against the self and against others and appear to stem from insecurity and feelings of guilt and inadequacy. In the drugged state the subjects appeared less disturbed by this conflict and had less need to harry themselves and others. They had a greater need for dominance, a desire for leadership. This ties in with the greater self-assurance demonstrated by other tests and with the increased awareness of acceptance by a love object found on this test.

It is interesting to note that these subjects showed no falling off in their awareness of illness and death or of restraint and imprisonment after smoking. The frequency of the latter concept was undoubtedly related to their status as prisoners, while the former ties in with the findings on the Free Association Test where the word "death" remained a disturbing factor even after marihuana had been smoked or ingested.

Findings on Women Subjects

As in the case with the men, when the female subject was under the influence of marihuana her basic personality structure did not change and only some relatively superficial emotional reactions were different. As a group, the women used in this study showed a somewhat constricted personality, and this constriction was not lessened when the subject was "high." The emotional reactions revealed in the Rorschach Test showed that the subjects in this particular group were primarily extraversive, and this remained unchanged after the administration of marihuana. Again, like the men, when under the influence of the drug the women lowered the achievement levels they set for themselves. However, they did not show any increased self-confidence as did the men, either by an increase in the number of words they claimed to know in the Loofbourrow Test or in their appraisal of themselves as indicated in the Downey Will-Temperament Test. In general, the women exhibited a loss of drive for participation in anything requiring effort. This is inferred from their performance in the Level of Aspiration Test, the Vocational Interest Blank, and the Binet Lines Test, as well as from their behavior.

Behavior During the Test Period of Subjects Under the Influence of Marihuana

The findings reported here have all been in terms of objective, quantitative measures. Some effects of the drug, observable during examinations, cannot be quantified but are nevertheless important to the understanding of the drug action. These effects were reflected in those reactions of the subjects which were not directly related to the test situation.

Behavior was somewhat different when the subject had ingested marihuana concentrate than it was when he had taken the drug in cigarette form. With pills gastro-intestinal disturbances were more pronounced and drowsiness and fatigue seemed greater and more enduring. Some individuals were so overcome by fatigue that they worked for a few seconds only, and then sat with their heads on the table. If spoken to, they made a great effort to do the work but rarely continued for very long. When summoned to take the test, especially towards the end of the day when they were almost invariably lying on their beds, the subjects were overcome with fatigue and were aroused only with the greatest difficulty. In some instances there was definite resentment of this disturbance and the impression was that only the presence of the police officer and all the implications in the prison set-up prevented a definite refusal to continue cooperatively. With both pills and cigarettes many of the men had difficulty in concentrating and maintaining a fixed goal. Subjects often stared vacantly for long periods and when addressed came back to the test with a start. Many burst into uncontrollable laughter over a test which in their undrugged state had evoked no merriment. This laughter frequently affected the entire group and most markedly those who had been given marihuana.

The behavior of the user and non-user with marihuana cigarettes was somewhat different. The user was pleasantly excited at the thought of smoking, selected his cigarettes with the manner of a connoisseur, and criticized or praised the product offered him. His smoking took on something of a ritualistic ceremony and was done in a careful and prearranged fashion which varied slightly from individual to individual. In general the men first opened the end of the cigarette to examine the marihuana, then wet the "stick" by inserting it in their mouths to prevent the paper from burning too rapidly. When the cigarette was ignited the men took several short puffs, at the same time inhaling as much air as possible. This caused the tip of the "stick" to glow and resulted in a succession of low gasping sounds from the subject. The smoke was retained as long as possible, occasionally causing severe paroxysms of coughing. Although eager to be "high" the user was consistent in his fear of "blowing his top," and there was always a point beyond which no amount of talking or cajoling could make him continue smoking. As a rule, the user liked to smoke in company. He was generally satisfied if one friend, a "kick partner," could be with him. To this friend he would explain his thoughts and feelings which to the objective observer were very superficial. In trying to make a point, and usually a minor one at that, the user, when smoking, would talk on endlessly and soon lose his goal. He cracked many "jokes" which were uproariously funny to him. In some instances "leaping" or involuntary jerking of the arms, head, shoulders or legs occurred. The subject described his sensations as floating, leaping, rocking or most often as being "in the groove." He was obviously enjoying pleasant physical sensations and wanted to be left to himself to lie on his bed, listen to soft music and dream or carry on "deep" conversations. The test questions were frequently called a "bring down" in that they forced the subject to face reality and abandon his pleasurable feelings. Several subjects concurred in describing part of their drug experience as comparable to the twilight state between sleeping and waking in which the individual floats pleasantly and does not allow outside stimuli to impinge. Just as strong extraneous sensations will bring the sleeper face to face with reality, so the insistence of the examiner that the subject perform certain tasks served to destroy his general feeling of well-being. Aside from the test situation any unpleasant circumstances can serve as a "bring down." This "bring down" apparently only results in destroying the subject's pleasure but cannot do away with the disadvantageous effect on intellectual functioning.

When testing was completed the subject generally lay on his bed and dozed or listened to the radio. His drowsiness persisted for many hours.

Most non-users approached the smoking with apprehension. They were instructed by the users in the art of lighting and inhaling, but they rarely cooperated to the fullest extent, though this was undoubtedly unconscious on their part.

The effects of marihuana on the non-users were variable. A few of them enjoyed the results so much that they claimed they would continue to smoke whenever they had a chance. They described such sensations as "lying in fur," and "floating in space." Some became acutely nauseous and could not continue with their work, while others experienced little or no change in feeling, undoubtedly because they never smoked correctly.

When the subjects were "high," particularly in the case of the non-user, there was a general loss of inhibition and lessening of many social restraints which had previously been exercised. Thus, all the men talked much more freely, confronted each other more directly, and manifested a state of well-being at times amounting to euphoria. They were much more confiding, talked spontaneously about love and sexual affairs, and in two instances exposed themselves and masturbated.

Although there was an undeniable increase in overt sex interest following the ingestion of marihuana, it seems probable that this interest was not the result of direct sexual stimulation but rather a manifestation of a falling off in inhibiting factors. This sex interest seems to have been due primarily to the fact that these men had been imprisoned for varying periods and had not had access to women. It is not at all certain that under free conditions or with different subjects this behavior would have been manifested. In any case, the behavior of these prisoners was more like that which any man deprived of sexual activity for a long period of time would display under a releasing stimulus and not at all like the behavior shown at marihuana "tea-pads."

Summary and Discussion

Under the influence of marihuana changes in personality as shown by alterations in test performance are slight. They are not statistically significant and indicate only tendencies or trends. Moreover, the drug effect is not always in proportion to the amount taken, nor are the changes consistently in one direction. In many instances the effect of small doses (2 cc.) or of marihuana cigarettes is the opposite of the effect of larger doses (5 cc.)*

The personality changes observed when the subject is under the influence of 2 cc. of marihuana or marihuana cigarettes demonstrate that the subject experiences some reduction in drive, less objectivity in evaluating situations, less aggression, more self-confidence and a generally more favorable attitude toward himself. These reactions can be ascribed to two main causes, namely, an increased feeling of relaxation and disinhibition and increased self-confidence. As the drug relaxes the subject, the restraints which he normally imposes on

*While sufficient experimentation has not been made to validate the finding, it should be noted that the personality changes produced by 2 cc. or marihuana cigarettes are almost always in agreement in contrast to the changes resulting from the ingestion of 5 cc. The 2 cc. dosage apparently more nearly approximates the amount a person would take if left to his own devices.

himself are loosened and he talks more freely than he does in his undrugged state. Things which under ordinary circumstances he would not speak about are now given expression. Metaphysical problems which in the undrugged state he would be unwilling to discuss, sexual ideas he would ordinarily hesitate to mention, jokes without point, are all part of the oral stream released by the marihuana.

At the same time that he verbalizes more freely, there is a reduction in the individual's critical faculty. This is probably due both to the intellectual confusion produced by the drug and to the less exacting attitude his feeling of relaxation induces. He holds himself less rigidly to the standards of his undrugged phase and does not drive himself to achieve. He is satisfied with himself and willing to accept himself as he is. This self-satisfaction undoubtedly helps produce the feeling of self-confidence which allows the subject to come out more freely in fields which he formerly avoided. This increased confidence expresses itself primarily through oral rather than physical channels. Physically the subject reports pleasant sensations of "drifting" and "floating" and he allows himself to become enveloped in a pleasant lassitude.

After the administration of larger doses of marihuana (5 cc.) the pleasurable sensations appear to be outweighed by concomitant feelings of anxiety and, in some cases, of physical distress, such as nausea. Under these circumstances, for many subjects there is little increase in confidence but rather heightened insecurity which precludes outgoing reactions and tends to evoke generally negativistic attitudes to most stimuli.

It is important to note that neither the ingestion of marihuana nor the smoking of marihuana cigarettes affects the basic outlook of the individual except in a very few instances and to a very slight degree. In general the subjects who are withdrawn and introversive stay that way, those who are outgoing remain so, and so on. Where changes occur the shift is so slight as to be negligible. In other words reactions which are natively alien to the individual cannot be induced by the ingestion or smoking of the drug.

Although in most instances the effects of the drug are the same for the user and the non-user, there are some differences both in kind and extent. Where the effects for the two groups are in the same direction they generally are more marked in the case of the non-user. This is not unexpected in view of the non-user's lack of habituation to the drug action. For the non user his present experience is a strange, even hazardous one, and the uncertainty and anxiety attendant upon this impairs the sense of well-being which the drug produces in the user. Thus the non-user frequently feels less secure when he is "high" than he does normally and is less well adjusted than he is in ordinary circumstances.

When the productions of the undrugged marihuana user are studied, certain personality traits which serve to differentiate him from the non-user and from the "average" individual can be discerned. As a group the marihuana users studied here were either inhibited emotionally or turned in on themselves, making little response to stimuli in the world about them. People with this type of personality generally have difficulty adjusting to others and are not at ease in social situations. This withdrawal from social contacts apparently finds little compensatory or sublimating activity elsewhere. These subjects did not have a desire or urge to occupy themselves creatively in a manner which might prove socially useful. They showed a tendency to drift along in passive fashion and gave a good portion of their attention to relatively unimportant matters. These men were poorly adjusted, lonely and insecure. As indicated by their history they seldom achieved good heterosexual adjustment.

Conclusions

1. Under the influence of marihuana the basic personality structure of the individual does not change but some of the more superficial aspects of his behavior show alteration.

2. With the use of marihuana the individual experiences increased feelings of relaxation, disinhibition and self-confidence.

3. The new feeling of self-confidence induced by the drug expresses itself primarily through oral rather than through physical activity. There is some indication of a diminution in physical activity.

4. The disinhibition which results from the use of marihuana releases what is latent in the individual's thoughts and emotions, but does not evoke responses which would be totally alien to him in his undrugged state.

5. Marihuana not only releases pleasant reactions but also feelings of anxiety.

6. Individuals with a limited capacity for affective experience and who have difficulty in making social contacts are more likely to resort to marihuana than those more capable of outgoing responses.

FAMILY AND COMMUNITY IDEOLOGIES

ADOLPH G. WOLTMANN, M.A.

At the outset of the study it seemed worth while to supplement the quantitative data by some qualitative procedures of the projective type which might throw light on the social reactions of the individuals who were being studied. One of the methods that has shown its possibilities, particularly in its use with children, is the play technique in which the individual is permitted to give free expression to some of his unconscious motivations in a way that is not immediately apparent to him. The limitation of this technique is the fact that it is highly interpretive, but it has the advantage of permitting observations of the subject's personality reactions in problem situations.

Such a study was accordingly carried out on 18 subjects in the early part of the investigation.

Method

Two situations were studied: one, subsequently to be referred to as the family set-up, in which toys were used to build an apartment or home, and another, subsequently to be known as the community set-up, in which a second variety of toys were used to construct a town setting.

THE FAMILY SET-UP

The equipment used in this part of the study consisted of a box of household toys of the type available in the ten-cent store, including beds, dressers, chairs, tables, sinks, a stove, a bathtub, a wash basin, a piano, lamps, flower boxes, a telephone, doll sets of a man, woman, boy, girl and maid, and, in addition, several small wooden slats which were intended to be used as room partitions.

The box of toys and materials was presented to the subject with the following directions: "Here are a number of toys which can be placed in such a manner that a house can be built from them. You are supposed to be this doll (man). Go ahead and build yourself a house or apartment. You may use as few or as many toys as you wish. You may also make believe you are a bachelor or a married man with or without a family."

The Community Set-up

In studying the community set-up the following items were employed: eighteen wooden houses, trees, cars, trucks, fire engines, an ambulance, a radio police car, a railroad train, airplanes, and numerous figures representing men, women and children from different walks of life. All these toys were handed to the subject at the same time with the instruction to build a town or city. As in the family set-up, no further help or suggestions were given.

The actual method of handling these materials allows for two approaches. In the free method the subject is encouraged to play with any toy and to create and act out any situation that the nature of the toy suggests to him. No help, clues or hints are given. In the controlled method either the subject is told to create a specific pattern or his responses and reactions to a predetermined particular situation are elicited. Both methods were used in this study.

After the subject had completed either his family or his community set-up and answered questions regarding certain situations about which the examiner had questioned him the following points were investigated: (1) subject's marital status, both real and assumed; (2) type of home he built for himself (number of rooms, type of furnishing); (3) subject's assumed occupation; (4) monthly income and rent which he posited; (5) his reaction to attempted burglary; (6) his reaction to his wife's and his own infidelity; and (7) the attitude he would take toward civic problems if given a position of responsibility such as mayor. In addition, the examiner appraised the subject's neatness and orderliness in his home and community set-up. The experiment was given first when the subject was undrugged and then when he was under the influence of marihuana.

Findings

Results were collated in terms of the type and frequency of responses to different situations both before and after taking marihuana and in terms of number of items (toys) employed in the set-up, as, for example, in the case of the home situation, the number of rooms the subject thought necessary for his apartment and the amount of rent he thought he ought to pay and its relation to the income he posited for himself; in the case of the community set-up, the number of times the subject provided for ambulances, firemen, and policemen; in the case of the subject's reaction to burglary, whether he took a passive or a resistant attitude toward the burglary and whether he assumed the burglar had absconded with most of the property and so on; in the case of his attitude toward his wife's adultery, whether he thought he ought to divorce her or try for reconciliation; and, when the subject was unfaithful, whether he thought his wife ought to forgive his delinquency.

In most cases comparisons between responses or reactions showed little difference in attitude before and after the ingestion of marihuana and therefore it would not to be too profitable in this short summary of the work to present all the data obtained. However, by way of illustrating the type of material procured, the following tables are given:

TABLE 36

Marital status of subjects

Marital status	In reality	During play	
		Without Marihuana	Under Marihuana
Married	4	14	13
Single	14	3	3
	18	17	16*

TABLE 37

Number of rooms planned for apartment during play

Number of Rooms	Number of subjects planning apartments	
	Without Marihuana	Under Marihuana
1	–	–
2	1	–
3	–	2
4	3	8
5	4	3
6	8	1
7	1	2
	17	16

*The differences between the number of subjects accounted for under different rubrics is due to the fact that occasionally a subject was not available for the test or retest experiment.

The majority of the patients, though unmarried in real life, assumed families and responsibilities in the play situation, and, in a free situation acted out family activities and ideologies.

These figures reveal that, on the average, the subjects when under the influence of the drug tended to build apartments with somewhat fewer rooms. The impression of the examiner was that this was due primarily to the subject's desire to get through with the task as quickly as possible in order to return to his room to rest and sleep.

TABLE 38

Frequency with which various toys were used during play

Toy	Number of times subjects used toys	
	Without Marihuana	Under Marihuana
Ambulance	14	7
Fire engine	6	6
Burglar	5	4
Police	5	2

A "make-believe" sickness or accident necessitating the use of an ambulance was the most frequently observed play pattern. When the subjects were under the influence of the drug the incidence of the ambulance and the police was considerably less than it was when they were in the undrugged state.

TABLE 39

Basic reactions to wife's adultery

Type of reaction	Number of subjects reacting	
	Without Marihuana	Under Marihuana
Passive	8	9
Aggressive	7	6
Not suspicious	2	1
	17	16

The most frequent form of passive reaction to his wife's infidelity was that the subject would pack up and leave home. The aggressive reactions consisted of ordering the wife out of the home in three instances, jailing the wife and lover in one instance, throwing the wife out in one instance, killing the lover but leaving the wife unmolested in one instance, and beating up the lover and leaving the wife unharmed in one instance.

The following are examples of subjects' reponses to the adultery situation. When he was facing the pretended situation before taking marihuana, one subject immediately left his house, borrowed money from his employer, and traveled to the West Coast. After he arrived there he proceeded to drink and in due time became a derelict on the Barbary Coast. When asked about his children he said, "That's closed with the rest of the chapter. Let her ardent lover support the children. I take on an assumed name. Others might get a divorce and custody of the children but in my case my home life would be a closed chapter." After the administration of marihuana he still showed a passive attitude, but, having assumed the role of a psychologist, he felt obliged to act accordingly. At first he considered divorce action but since that would deprive the children of a home, he finally forgave his wife. Then he stopped in his contemplations, looked at the examiner and said, "Why do I become altruistic? . . . That's beyond me . . . Maybe I become a martyr . . . I commit an act of martyrdom." Another subject, when in the undrugged condition, ordered his wife out of the house and later divorced her. In the drugged state customary procedures were reversed. The subject went to his parents and remain passively at home while his mother unsuccessfully tried to bring about a reconciliation.

TABLE 40

Final solution to the problem of wife's adultery

Solution	Number of subjects	
	Without Marihuana	Under Marihuana
Reconciliation	2	2
Separation	1	1
Divorce	7	5
Separation without legal advice	7	8
	17	16

The subject's attitude toward adultery did not change in the drugged state. The data in Table 40 illustrate the fact that ingestion of marihuana generally does not alter the subject's basic attitude.

TABLE 41

Attitude toward saloons, gambling, prostitution and marihuana

Attitude toward various civic problems		Number of subjects expressing attitudes	
		Without Marihuana	Under Marihuana
Saloons:	Approval	12	13
	Disapproval	2	1
Gambling:	Approval	4	4
	Disapproval	10	10
Prostitution:	Approval	9	8
	Disapproval	5	6
Marihuana:	Approval	4	8
	Disapproval	10	6

Practically all the subjects approved of saloons. Gambling was rejected because it deprives wives and children of money and leads to trouble. A heavy loser may try to recoup his losses through hold-ups, and fights and homicide may develop from quarrels. Prostitution was condoned by about 50 per cent of the subjects both before and after the ingestion of the drug, but the use of marihuana was frowned upon more often when the subject was undrugged than when he was in the drugged state.

Summary and Conclusions

Eighteen subjects who participated in the marihuana study were subjected to the play situation with the idea of seeing whether the pattern of play or the ideas investigated were materially altered in consequence of the ingestion of the marihuana. Among the ideologies which were appraised were: (1) attitude toward family set-up; (2) attitude toward different occupations; (3) attitude toward income; (4) attitude toward situations ordinarily calling for aggression, namely an attempted burglary of his home and sexual infidelity on the part of his wife; (5) attitude toward authority.

In general the subject's attitude toward family and community ideologies as manifested in play did not change markedly as a result of the ingestion of marihuana. The subjects (in play) were not intolerant of infidelity or aggressive toward lawbreakers either before or after the ingestion of marihuana. On the whole the initial passive reactions already observed in other parts of the study were likewise observed in the play situation experiment. The only very definite change as a result of the ingestion of marihuana was in their attitude toward the drug itself. Without marihuana only 4 out of 14 subjects said they would tolerate the sale of marihuana while after ingestion 8 of them were in favor of this.

Another significant manifestation in the play situation pertains to the construction of the community set-up. In general the community was less orderly and well organized when the subjects had had marihuana. It is probable that this poor organization may be ascribed to the generally indifferent attitude and lack of motor coordination already observed in the more controlled studies.

On the whole, the experiment with play technique gave less information as to the effect of marihuana on subjects than had been hoped for. This may have been due to the incompleteness of the method employed or possibly to the fact that this technique is designed to give data about the basic personality of the individual rather than such alterations in it as might be caused by pharmacological agents.

Comparison Between Users and Non-Users from the Standpoint of Mental and Physical Deterioration

A careful testing of the motor and sensory functions of the nervous system was included in the general physical examination of each subject. Of motor functions, reflex activity and muscular response and coordination were determined; of sensory functions, perception of touch, pain and temperature stimuli; of specialized functions, taste, hearing and vision. In the eye, the corneal and light reflexes were tested and a retinal examination was made. In this neurological examination no pathological conditions were found in any of the subjects.

In the psychiatric examination attention was paid to general intelligence and knowledge in relation to the subject's background, to relevancy of talk in conversation, to orientation as to time, place and situation, to memory of past and recent events, to ability in simple arithmetic, to judgment in reaching decisions, and to the presence of abnormal mental content shown by delusions, hallucinations, obsessions, and ideas of persecution. There was no evidence of disordered cerebral functioning in any of the group.

As would be expected, differences in grades of intelligence and in orderliness in thinking and reasoning were noticeable. The Bellevue Adult Intelligence Test was administered to a total of 60 male subjects, 40 marihuana users and 20 non-users. The average I.Q. for the user group was 96.7, range 70 to 124, and for the non-user group the average I.Q. was 104.5, range 93 to 114. Both groups may therefore be classified as of average intelligence.

When analyzed according to racial distribution the two groups were even better equated intellectually than the total results indicate. For the 28 white subjects examined (13 users and 15 non-users), the average I.Q. for the users was 106.1, range 77 to 124, and for the non-users the average I.Q. was 106.3, range 96 to 114. There were 24 Negro subjects, 19 users and 5 non-users. The average I.Q. for the users was 92.6, range 70 to 112, while for the non-users the average I.Q. was 98.8, range 93 to 101. Although the non-users averaged 6.2 points higher than the users, it must be taken into account that the number of Negro non-users tested was small. In any event, the disparity in results would not be considered significant. The average I.Q. of the 8 Puerto Rican users was 91.0, range 72 to 100.

Reports on mental deterioration due to toxic, organic or psychotic factors as given in the literature, reveal that in such cases the individual scores on the Bellevue Adult Intelligence Test show marked irregularity, depending upon the functions involved in the deteriorative process. As a group, the marihuana users tested in this study showed very even functioning, and what little irregularity occurred can be explained on the basis of language and racial factors.

The physical and psychiatric examinations were of a qualitative rather than a quantitative nature. In the special examinations and tests of organ and system function, quantitative measurements were obtained. Findings in 17 marihuana users are given in Table 42. These subjects were selected for the reason that they had smoked marihuana for the longest period of time. The figures for years of usage and number of cigarettes smoked daily are taken from each subject's statement.

It is seen from Table 42 that the marihuana users, accustomed to daily smoking for a period of from two and a half to sixteen years, showed no abnormal system functioning which would differentiate them from the non-users.

There is definite evidence in this study that the marihuana users were not inferior in intelligence to the general population and that they had suffered no mental or physical deterioration as a result of their use of the drug.

TABLE 42

Laboratory findings on seventeen marihuana users

Subject	Years of usage	Number of cigarettes per day	Pulse rate per min.	Blood pressure	Vital capacity (in L.)	Hemo-globin %	Red blood cells	White blood cells	Urea nitrogen (mg. %)	Calcium (mg. %)	Phos-phorus (mg. %)	Sugar (mg. %)	P.S.P. Excre-tion (%)	Basal Me-tabo-lism
M.R.	16	2–4	80	120/80	3.7	85	5,130,000	13,800	24.9	—	—	89	40	2
J.P.	14	10–15	84	130/88	3.2	85	6,500,000	7,900	11	—	—	81	51	−15
C.D.	13	2	90	126/82	4.5	85	4,600,000	14,850	12.6	—	—	85	—	−12
M.G.	11	18	92	110/80	3.5	90	5,360,000	9,100	16.2	—	—	97	55	− 2
O.D.	10	2	60	118/76	4.8	92	4,600,000	12,400	8.5	10.2	3.5	87.5	65	4
F.W.	10	2–3	88	120/86	2.8	95	4,590,000	12,700	14.5	—	—	99	47	−11
F.G.	8	12	68	120/86	4.2	97	4,400,000	7,400	11.5	11.4	2.9	85	52	−12
C.B.	8	8	92	130/78	4.0	85	4,790,000	10,700	11	—	—	83	65	− 7

W.R.	8	5	64	100/62	3.1	85	5,110,000	8,200	13.6	11.2	5.5	60	40	−17
R.T.	6	2–6	76	98/62	3.6	95	5,400,000	8,400	13.1	11.1	3.5	75	51	− 7
W.C.	6	8–9	80	130/105	3.1	70	5,600,000	14,500	13	—	—	55	55	− 6
J.B.	5	2	68	104/82	4.1	90	4,900,000	10,200	10.7	—	—	88	37.5	− 4
A.B.	5	5	120	120/74	3.9	93	4,480,000	9,400	10.8	10.7	3.1	87.5	45	− 5
J.N.	5	10–12	62	100/58	3.1	90	5,200,000	7,500	9.7	—	—	91	61	−20
C.J.	5	10	74	110/85	4.1	90	6,050,000	8,000	13.2	—	—	84.5	45	4
J.H.	4	7	74	130/70	3.4	90	4,360,000	10,500	14.4	—	—	98	57	−13
B.W.	2½	10	88	135/75	4.7	80	6,000,000	9,100	12.2	—	—	73	60	−22

Addiction and Tolerance

A drug addiction is characterized by a compelling urge to use the drug for the prevention or relief of distressing mental and physical disturbances which occur when the necessary dose is delayed or omitted. A drug habit is also characterized by an urge to use the drug, but this is not compelling. The abstinence symptoms, which are expressions of nervous states, are not particularly distressing and do not occur as long as the person's attention is placed on other matters.

Drug tolerance in the narrower sense used here means that larger doses than those originally used are required to bring about the effects desired by the subject. In the case of morphine, tolerance develops because of addiction, but in other instances tolerance may be present without addiction and addiction without tolerance. When both are present the matter takes on greater importance because of the extremes to which the addict goes to obtain the drug constantly and in increasing quantities.

As our group of subjects included 48 users of marihuana, opportunity was afforded for some conclusions concerning marihuana addiction and tolerance. Practically all of our group of users stated that they could and often did voluntarily stop the smoking for a time without any undue disturbance from the deprivation. In the sociologic study reported by Dr. Shoenfeld it was found that smokers had no compelling urge for marihuana. If "reefers" were not readily available there was no special effort made to obtain them from known sources of supply. Dr. Walter Bromberg, Psychiatrist-in-Charge, Psychiatric Clinic, Court of General Sessions in New York, states: "The fact that offenders brought up on marihuana charges do not request medical treatment on their incarceration (with its cessation of drug supply) argues for the absence of withdrawal symptoms."[(1)] From interviews with several hundred marihuana users he concludes that true addiction was absent.

The evidence submitted here warrants the conclusion that as far as New York City is concerned true addiction to marihuana does not occur.

The evidence concerning acquired tolerance is less clear-cut. Tolerance develops during the periods when the drug is being taken and

(1) Bromberg, W. Marihuana: a psychiatric study. J.A.M.A. 113:4, 1939.

accounts for the necessity of increasing the dosage to bring about the desired effects. How long the tolerance persists after the drug administration is stopped has not been definitely established in any instance.

The statements of marihuana usage and time since stoppage given by eight of our subjects are summarized in Table 43.

TABLE 43

History of marihuana use among eight subjects

Subjects	Years of Usage	Number of Cigarettes Smoked Daily	Period of Deprivation
J. B.	5	5	2 weeks
W. C.	5	8	4 weeks
J. P.	14	10	7 weeks
A. B.	5	5	2 months
J. H.	4	7	2 months
F. G.	8	10	2½ months
O. D.	10	2	7 months
C. B.	8	6	2 years

On one or more of the numerous occasions on which marihuana was administered each of these subjects received what was considered a minimal effective dose. One (J.B.) was given 1 cc., another (A.B.) 3 cc., the others 2 cc. In all instances the customary physical effects, conjunctival injection, dilated and sluggishly reacting pupils, tremors and ataxia, were observed. With these doses the subjects also experienced the sensation described as "high." The only conclusion warranted here is that if acquired tolerance does occur it persists for a limited period only.

Further evidence, though indirect, was brought out by Dr. Shoenfeld's investigation and by personal interviews with our 48 users. There is agreement in the statements that among users the smoking of one or two cigarettes is sufficient to bring on the effect known as "high." When this state is reached the user will not continue smoking for fear of becoming "too high." When the desired effects have passed off and the smoker has "come down," smoking one cigarette brings the "high" effect on again. This could not be the case had a steadily increasing tolerance developed.

The evidence available then—the absence of any compelling urge to use the drug, the absence of any distressing abstinence symptoms, the statements that no increase in dosage is required to repeat the desired effect in users—justifies the conclusion that neither true addiction nor tolerance is found in marihuana users. The continuation and the frequency of usage of marihuana, as in the case of many other habit-forming substances, depend on the easily controlled desires for its pleasurable effects.

Possible Therapeutic Applications

If a drug has well-marked pharmacological actions and low toxicity, as appears to be the case with marihuana, a consideration of special interest is its possible therapeutic application. In the older clinical literature marihuana was recommended for use in a wide variety of disorders, but in recent years it has almost disappeared from the materia medica and it was dropped from the United States Pharmacopeia twenty years ago.

In view of the laboratory and clinical findings obtained in this study the question of the therapeutic possibilities of the drug was considered. Marihuana possesses two qualities which suggest that it might have useful actions in man. The first is the typical euphoria-producing action which might be applicable in the treatment of various types of mental depression; the second is the rather unique property which results in the stimulation of appetite. In the light of this evidence and in view of the fact that there is a lack of any substantial indication of dependence on the drug, it was reasoned that marihuana might be useful in alleviating the withdrawal symptoms in drug addicts.

At the Riker's Island Penitentiary observations were made on 56 inmates who were addicted to morphine or heroin. Two groups were selected, the addicts in each being matched with those in the other group as to age, physical condition, duration and intensity of habit, and number of previous attempts at cure. The subjects in one group received no treatment or were given Magendie's solution according to the usual hospital regimen, while those in the other group were treated with 15 mg. of tetrahydrocannabinol three times daily with or without placebo (subcutaneous water injection). An attempt was made to evaluate the severity of the withdrawal signs and symptoms. The impression was gained that those who received tetrahydrocannabinol had less severe withdrawal symptoms and left the hospital at the end of the treatment period in better condition than those who received no treatment or who were treated with Magendie's solution. The ones in the former group maintained their appetite and in some cases actually gained weight during the withdrawal period.

Since psychological factors play a large part in the withdrawal symptoms of at least a certain proportion of morphine addicts, there are grounds for the assumption that a drug having the properties of marihuana might be of aid in alleviating mental distress during the withdrawal period. However, the studies here described were not sufficiently complete to establish the value of such treatment, and before conclusions can be drawn the problem must be investigated under completely controlled conditions.

PHARMACOLOGICAL STUDY †

S. LOEWE, M.D.*

I. The Relationship Between Structure and Activity and the Significance of Coordinated Pharmacological and Chemical Investigations As Applied to Marihuana

In studying the biological activity of marihuana, the active principles of which have not been identified, one deals with a mixture of uncertain composition. The crude preparations employed in the past revealed a broad spectrum of pharmacological qualities, based upon the pharmacological actions and effects of all the constituents present. Each effect may be attributed to one or another of the numerous components of the complex mixture, or all the effects may be due to only one of a large number of components present.

In the case of marihuana this difficult situation is testified to by the long history of unsuccessful efforts. When our studies began (1937), the closest approach to the isolation of an active principle from marihuana was probably the preparation of a substance with rather moderate marihuana activity by Bergel and Wagner.[22] This substance was not isolated from marihuana but obtained by chemical manipulation *in vitro*, and its chemical nature was only partially known. Even the most recent attempts to review our knowledge of the chemical nature of the active principle[25, 65] were mainly concerned with compounds of marihuana which we now know to be inactive.

In the search for the unknown active principle every step of the fractionation of the raw material by the chemist requires parallel pharmacological studies to distinguish between the effective and ineffective fractions, and to indicate how the various effects have been influenced by the chemical procedure. "In all probability the chemical constitution of this unique substance is not going to be definitely recognized until there is a coordinated investigative program in which the chemical alterations are guided directly by accurate measurements of physiological activity." This is the closing sentence of Walton's book[65] which reviews the period of unsuccessful endeavor to isolate the active principles of marihuana.

---

†From the Department of Pharmacology, Cornell University Medical College.

*Part of the experimental work here reported was conducted in collaboration with W. Modell.

The immediate need would be satisfied by a program of coordinated endeavor by chemical and pharmacological laboratories leading to the isolation of the unknown active substance. Chemical synthesis is necessary only in so far as it is desirable to complete the identification of the natural substance by its synthesis *in vitro*. However, chemical synthesis is important in a wider sense, namely, to bring the pharmacological and chemical properties of the new substance into accord with our conceptions of the basis of biological activity in general, and to broaden these conceptions by adding information on how and why biological activity varies with variations in chemical structure. Contributions to this general problem of the relationship between structure and activity, which has long interested the chemist and the biologist, can only be expected from their coordinated efforts.

It was due to the foresight of the United States Bureau of Narcotics and the Narcotics Laboratory of the United States Treasury Department that the teamwork for the realization of this program was put into effect. Inaugurated by Dr. H. J. Anslinger, Commissioner of Narcotics, the teamwork resulted from the coordinated investigations of three groups: the large scale preparatory and analytical work by Dr. H. J. Wollner, Dr. J. R. Matchett, et al. in Washington, D. C., associated with work in the United States Department of Agriculture, the analytical and synthetic research by Dr. R. Adams et al. in the Department of Chemistry, University of Illinois, and the pharmacological investigations of the author who, after an initial period of marihuana work in the Montefiore Hospital Laboratory of the Medical Division, enjoyed the hospitality of Cornell University Medical College, with the invaluable support and advice of Dr. McKeen Cattell and the collaboration of Dr. Walter Modell. In its major parts, the present survey of the pharmacology of marihuana deals with the results of this teamwork.*

II. Sources of Drugs With Marihuana Activity

The interest in marihuana exhibited by so many branches of the medical and social sciences is due to its specific effect upon the higher cerebral functions, including its psychic action, and to its wide use

* This report was completed in February 1942. Shortly thereafter the chemical aspects were reviewed by R. Adams in his Harvey Lecture.[72] Subsequent progress has been given consideration mainly in footnotes and in an addendum to the bibliography. Nov. 1943.

for the purpose of producing euphoria and mental relaxation. These effects may be grouped under the term marihuana activity.

Materials with marihuana activity have been widely used in the past in many parts of the world, in a great variety of preparations and under a great variety of names. It is not the purpose of this report to go into details of the history, the origin or the nomenclature of all these sources of marihuana activity. Information on these questions and on the state of our knowledge of marihuana up to 1938, which covers the period before the isolation of the active principles, will be found in Walton's excellent book which includes a full bibliography.[65] A botanical description with instructive illustrations will be found in a pamphlet edited by the United States Treasury Department.[62]

The numerous preparations having marihuana activity are all obtained from members of the *Cannabinaceae* family. These are usually distinguished from the common hemp by differences in their geographical origin; for example, plants with marihuana activity are found in the Americas ["Cannabis Americana" in the United States of America and Mexico ("marihuana," "marijuana") and in Brazil ("maconha")], as well as in Africa and Asia ["Cannabis indica," in India ("bhanga," "ganja"), Arabia and Persia ("hashish," mainly designating the resin), China ("Cannabis sinensis," "Ma"), North and West Africa ("diamba," "riamba") and South Africa ("dakha")], and also in Italy and Roumania.

Two circumstances have contributed to a breakdown of botanical distinctions: 1) The demonstration of marihuana activity in hemp weeds from a moderate climate, as for instance in plants grown on vacant lots in the vicinity of New York City. 2) The investigations underlying the inclusion of marihuana in the Federal Tax Legislation of August 2, 1937. Since then it has been generally acknowledged that the source of all preparations with marihuana activity is Cannabis sativa Linn., the common hemp.

The main source of marihuana preparations is the tops of female plants at or shortly after the peak of the period of flowering. The flowering female tops are especially rich in resinous exudate. The amount of this exudate is sometimes increased by special measures such as removal of male plants from the fields, early cutting of larger leaves, and dwarfing the entire plant. Where the exudation is plentiful, preparations are made up from the resin by beating, kneading and pressing after freeing the harvested tops from leaves, stalks and twigs. This resinous material is used by preference in Oriental countries and is variously prepared for smoking, chewing, eating or even snuffing. However, the entire leaf is sometimes used for preparing potions or confections, or for preparing cigarettes with or without added tobacco. The resin itself can also be collected in the field by dusting, beating, scraping or rubbing it from tops, leaves, stalks and twigs. Seeds are present as additional components in some preparations, particularly confections, and there are indications that they are sometimes used alone in crushed form.

Many misinterpretations regarding the potency of products obtained from various hemps, as well as from various parts of the plant, can now be attributed to a pharmacognostic error, namely, the use of a chemical reaction which, while sufficiently specific for the hemp herb, cannot be attributed to the active components. According to present opinion, the marihuana activity is related to the oil content. It is for this reason that significance is attached to the yield of extractives obtained with the aid of organic solvents. According to the literature these extractives amount to 11-26 per cent (generally about 12 per cent) of the herb in Oriental hemp, 6-12 per cent in African and 6-10 per cent in American hemp, and to about 40 per cent of the resin collected from Oriental hemp. Such data usually refer to alcoholic extracts; the yields in extractives (not in active principles) are from 15 to 50 per cent lower when ethyl ether is employed, and 25 per cent (or in the case of resin from 25 to 50 per cent) lower with petroleum ether.

Variations in the content of resinous and oily extractives more or less parallel the content of active principles and are ascribed to differences in climate and soil. Only by the application of a uniform method for the extraction of the active components and the development of a quantitative biological test for potency was it established that, notwithstanding the now acknowledged species uniformity, there are genotypic factors governing the content of active principles. A study of this problem was conducted in collaboration with the Narcotics Laboratory of the Treasury Department and the Department of Agriculture. The scope was to examine marihuana activity in hemp plants grown for a number of generations on the same soil (Arlington, Virginia) from seeds of very different geographical origin. Figures obtained with our ataxia method of bioassay in the dog (and, for comparison, with B. B. Robinson's goldfish test[56]) are presented in Table 49, preparations 4, 5, 6 and 9. They show that, after three generations, Tunisian hemp is still 4, 6 and 8.7 times as potent as a Wisconsin, a Kentucky, and a Manchurian hemp respectively; thus the original differences in activity were maintained over three generations of growth under uniform circumstances of climate and soil. Such hereditary differences in the capacity of producing active substances independently of environmental influences signify that varieties of Cannabis sativa can be distinguished not only on the basis of morphological characteristics but also on the basis of chemical criteria.

The resin, the major source of marihuana active principles, is a surface excretion, mainly of the tops and the leaves, and it is frequently assumed that it has a protective function against the drying influence of environmental heat. Indication of a wider distribution is seen in the fact that the seeds are also utilized by marihuana users. Whether or not they contain active components was a matter of dispute. We endeavored therefore to determine the biological activity of hemp seeds by means of the ataxia test in the dog. Due to the abundance of fatty substances, the active materials in extracts prepared by the Narcotics Laboratory (J. R. Matchett) by means of organic solvents were too dilute to give a definite response. However, in concentrates prepared by saponifying the fatty extracts and isolating the nonsaponifiable fraction, the presence of active substances was demonstrated beyond doubt.[53] The percentage of active components was low in comparison with that of resins or extracts from flowering tops and even with that of the dried tops themselves. The quantity of the nonsaponifiable fraction obtained from 675 Gm. of seeds was 4 Gm., with a potency of 0.035, that is, if the active substance is assumed to be of the same potency as that in the tops, the fraction contained about 95 per cent of inert nonsaponifiable materials. The figures indicate, furthermore, that if the nonsaponifiable fraction represented all the active components in the seeds, the potency of the seeds was only 1/100 that of dry hemp. However, it is obvious that, due to losses of various kinds during the extraction and saponification, these tests may have yielded only minimum figures. It is clear that the seeds must also be taken into account as a source of marihuana.

As to the problem of distribution of active components over the different parts of the hemp plant, it should be pointed out that the use of the chemical reaction (Beam's color test) is responsible for the assumption of an almost ubiquitous distribution of the active components throughout the entire plant and of their presence at all periods of the life span of the plant. However, Bouquet[26] found plants up to four months old exempt from this rule, that is, they were Beam-negative. In an extensive and painstaking statistical analysis of a great variety of hemps by the Narcotics Laboratory and the Department of Agriculture,[52, 57, 61, 63] the chemical test was found to be positive in the extracts from an overwhelming majority of plants with no marked difference between earlier and later phases of development. Some of these and a number of additional extracts which had been subjected to the Beam test were bioassayed on dogs in our laboratory with the following results:

TABLE 44

Hemp Origin	Grown in	Alkaline Beam Test	Physiological Activity
Minnesota	Minnesota	negative	active
Minnesota	Minnesota	negative	active
(Extract from crop standing 3½ years in the stack)			
Minnesota	Minnesota	feeble	active
(Extract from crop standing 3½ years in the stack)			
Manchuria	Arlington, Va.	weak	active
Roumania	Arlington, Va.	very strong	very low potency

These tests gave the first indication that potency and color reaction can be significantly divergent. It will be seen in a later part of this report that the alkaline Beam test is not an indicator for any substance having marihuana activity. Thus, the proposition holds true that when a very complex mixture exhibits a characteristic chemical and a characteristic biological quality, it is not likely that these two qualities are determined by one and the same substance out of the many in the mixture. It is true, however, that the Beam-positive substance, although biologically inert, is closely related to that part of the metabolic function of the hemp plant which is responsible for the production of active substances (see page 163). A positive Beam test is therefore indicative of substances chemically affiliated with the active principles and shows, irrespective of whether they may be precursors of the active principle or transformation products, that the

TABLE 45

Lethal doses of marihuana

Animal	Preparation	Administration	Lethal dose (Mg./Kg.)	Remarks
Frog	"Standard Extract"	Subcutaneously	7500	"Deep narcosis or death" [39]
Albino mouse	Crude Extractives from Hashish	Intraperitoneally	1600	Wiechowski [67]
Albino mouse	Hashish Resin	Intraperitoneally	500	Balozet [21]
Rat	American Fluid Extract	Intraperitoneally	6–700	Walton [66]
Guinea-pig	American Fluid Extract	Intraperitoneally	250	Walton [66]
Rabbit	American Fluid Extract	Intravenously	430	Loewe (unpublished)
Dog	American Fluid Extract	Intravenously	1700	Hare [41]
Dog	American Fluid Extract	Intravenously	>5400	Houghton and Hamilton [42]

plant is—or was—ready to produce active substances. In this sense the Beam test, although it by no means proves that the active principles are generally distributed, does show that substances chemically related to the active principles are present in many parts of the plant and that they occur in the early phases of development, from the seed stage on.

This raises the question of whether those parts of the plants that are utilized by various fiber industries are also to be considered as sources of active principles. These parts are the stalks of the fully developed plant. For all purposes of fiber utilization the stalks are freed from nonfibrous components by mechanical, biological and chemical procedures. Among the latter, bleaching with strong oxidants is the most destructive treatment regularly applied. The problem of whether fiber products of the hemp may still serve as a source of marihuana activity was studied in a few experiments in collaboration with the Narcotics Laboratory. Fibers and hurds from an early stage in the manufacturing process were extracted with organic solvents and the extracts subjected to biological examination. In none of these extracts, not even with doses equivalent to large amounts of the original material, was it possible to demonstrate the presence of activity. In addition, the author also prepared extracts from materials from a later stage in the manufacturing process, namely, the pulp employed for the manufacture of certain papers from hemp fibers. The yield in extractives from this material was even less than that from unprepared fibers or hurds, and even in high dosage none of these extracts elicited signs of marihuana action.

III. The Pharmacological Actions of Marihuana

All the earlier studies on the physiological effects of hemp were conducted with relatively crude materials, since none of the active principles had been isolated or identified. The result was an unbalanced picture of the composite pharmacological activity of this mixture, since preparations of differing composition and source were employed for those studies. The discussion of marihuana effects will be limited to those aspects of the composite picture which can be attributed to the principles isolated in the course of the present work or which had been assumed in previous studies to be characteristic of the chief active principles.

Lethality

Data on the lethal effect of crude drug preparations have very little significance. This is illustrated in Table 45, in which the more important data on marihuana are assembled.

Gastro-intestinal Symptoms

Retching and vomiting are frequent symptoms. They occur irregularly, as does diarrhea, but they may be produced by both crude extracts and pure substances, and are observed following both enteral and parenteral administration. In the majority of cases, irrespective of the dose, these effects occur after a considerable period of latency. However, this period (twenty to one hundred minutes) is not longer after intravenous injection, and therefore the action is systemic and probably central.

Circulatory Symptoms

In the literature a number of effects more or less related to the circulatory system have been attributed to marihuana. For example, the extensive data reported by Marx and Eckhardt[51] show a striking decrease in pulse rate. An interpretation of this observation is suggested by the authors' report that all their dogs showed an initial period of excitation and great motor hyperactivity (probably due to the fact that the animals were allowed freedom in the observation room and that the decreasing pulse rate returned to normal "parallel to ebbing of the excitation phase"). The question of whether alterations in pulse rate and other circulatory functions are consistent symptoms related to specific marihuana actions can be answered only through the study of purified preparations. Some experimental findings bearing on this problem will be reported in the section on the active principles (page 193).

Motor Symptoms

Fibrillary tremors are frequently observed in animals at the same time as the other motor disturbance, incoordination. There are other indications that the fibrillary tremor is a symptom closely correlated with the ataxia.

Ataxia which, since 1844 or earlier,[49] has been recognized as a specific symptom of marihuana action, is due to loss of normal motor coordination. It is best displayed in the dog, but is also seen in cats, and with less characteristic manifestations in rabbits and rhesus monkeys. Manifestations of the loss in coordination of muscular activity are (I) an almost imperceptible swaying in the upright position; (II) more pronounced swaying both sideways and along the longitudinal axis of the body; (III) swaying and rocking of an intensity such that the point of gravity may occasionally shift markedly forward or backward; (IV) occasional loss of balance resulting in stumbling or falling; (V) loss of the capacity to maintain the upright position and complete inability to regain it from a recumbent position. The numbers in parentheses are used (Walton et al.[66]) to designate different grades of ataxia.

Ataxia can best be observed in animals favoring an upright position. This is perhaps the main reason why the dog is preferred and why dogs with long legs are the most suitable test animals.

That the intensity of effect progresses as a function of increasing doses has been denied by some authors. These denials are doubtless due to a prominent feature of all ataxia effects, namely, that up to the highest grades they can be abolished for a varying period of time by external stimuli. In lower grades of ataxia moderate stimuli are sufficient, but even the highest grades can be abolished. A prostrate animal may be aroused from a state of deep apathy. Persistent adequate stimuli may prevent the manifestations of ataxia for the entire duration of drug action. In well-calibrated animals giving a quantitatively reproducible response to marihuana, the strongly antagonistic effect of stimuli such as exposure to cool, stormy and windy weather, mating or delivery, was apparent. An opinion on the reproducibility of ataxia symptoms and on the correlation between dosage and intensity of symptoms can be formed only when the worker is well acquainted with the animal and its reaction to marihuana.

Details of the manifestations of motor incoordination in the dog, not mentioned here, have been extensively described by others. In short, the effect in the dog resembles in all its main features and in numerous details the syndrome of cerebellar ataxia produced in the dog by extirpation of the cerebellum and in man resulting from cerebellar lesions.

Peripheral Nervous Symptoms

Two consistent sensory effects of marihuana are scratching and corneal anesthesia. Scratching is best manifested in dogs. It is observed only when doses large enough to produce ataxia are given, but it usually appears before the symptoms of ataxia. It is less pronounced during the higher degrees of ataxia, and this may be one reason why it is not an absolutely consistent sign of marihuana action. The sign is an intensification of the normal scratch reflex of the dog and has all its features. In some instances, particularly at the onset of strong ataxia action, it is performed by circling around the longitudinal axis of the body as if the scratching were elicited by an itching on the head. It is not known whether this symptom is due to a sensory action of the drug, that is, to primary paresthesia, or to stimulation of central or efferent parts of the scratch reflexes.

The corneal anesthesia first described by Gayer[38] is not manifested in the dog but is observed in rabbits, and, according to some authors, also in the cat and the mouse. We[47] observed varying but inconclusive intensities of corneal anesthesia in mice to which a combination of a dose of marihuana with a threshold hypnotic dose of a barbiturate (pernoston) had been administered. The incidence of corneal anesthesia was greater in these animals than in those which had been given the same threshold dose of pernoston alone, whereas corneal anesthesia was absent in all animals treated with marihuana alone.

Corneal anesthesia was usually studied in rabbits after intravenous administration of the drug.* The effect is manifested by partial or complete abolition of the wink reflex of the three eyelids of the rabbit in response to a touch stimulus applied to the cornea. The areflexia may be complete or incomplete according to the intensity and localization of the stimulus and according to the dose of the drug. In all these features the marihuana effect is very similar to the corneal anesthesia produced by the application of a local anesthetic. However, the corneal anesthesia effect of marihuana is unique in that it is produced only by systemic action of the drug. The effectiveness of marihuana is much lower after oral than after intravenous

* Gayer[38] recommended acetone as a solvent for intravenous injection. In our own studies on the intravenous toxicity of some organic solvents in the rabbit, the lethal dose of acetone was markedly lower (about 0.5 cc. per Kg.) than that of ethanol. Therefore, we prefer ethanol as the vehicle for intravenous injection of resinous or oily marihuana substances. Later we found propylene glycol to be a much superior vehicle.

administration. According to Gayer,[38] the minimum effective dose is 0.3 Gm. per Kg. intravenously, expressed in equivalents of dry hemp herb, but ten times this amount is required orally.

A significant difference between the corneal areflexias from systemic marihuana action and from local action of drugs of the cocaine group, which is not mentioned in the literature, is the failure of marihuana to prevent responses from more distant parts of the body. When the lid response is completely abolished by the influence of marihuana, reflex reactions of the neck muscles may persist.* This singular syndrome of abolition of the lid reflex and an undiminished reflex response of other muscles may indicate that the influence of marihuana upon those reflexes is brought about by a mechanism other than the loss of peripheral sensory perception.

Mydriasis, either by peripheral or by central action, is often mentioned as a sign of marihuana action in humans as well as in laboratory animals. According to Walton,[66] dilatation of the pupil is not a consistent phenomenon in the laboratory experiment. Neither in the rabbit nor in the dog or cat have we been able to note any regularity in the appearance of mydriasis.

Central Nervous Symptoms

Numerous attempts to demonstrate hypnotic and sedative effects in various species of animals led to the trial of marihuana preparations to induce sleep and to decrease various forms of nervous excitation. Experiments on lower animals in which a decrease in motility results from a general paralyzing action have been thought to represent a hypnotic action. This group of experiments contains studies on daphnia (Viehover[64]), on goldfish (Robinson[56]), on frogs (Balozet[31]) and on other forms. Among higher animals, the cat is reported to show a "depressed behavior" and a general weakening of reflexes. Decreasing motility in the dog due to motor ataxia may be interpreted as "sleep" by a superficial observer. A central depressant action of marihuana has been described in horses and recommended for therapeutic purposes in veterinary medicine; however, in spite of this "depressant action," marihuana has been used as an illegal stimulant for race horses.

Another approach to the question of the hypnotic influence of marihuana is based upon the consideration that a weak hypnotic

* Loewe and Modell, unpublished.

action can be increased by combination with low doses of real hypnotics. The existence of such an hypnotic action was concluded by Buergi[28] from experiments on synergism in rabbits; they have not been confirmed, and their significance for the marihuana problem is thrown in doubt by the fact that Buergi reported the same effects with aqueous extracts which we now know contain neither specific nor "hypnotic" principles.[54] Attempts to demonstrate synergism in albino mice[47, 48] with a number of barbiturates were unsuccessful except for one bromine-containing barbiturate, pernoston. The hypnotic effect of a threshold dose of pernoston was markedly and regularly prolonged in groups of mice. A similar increase in effect was obtained by pernoston alone when the dose was increased by only 10 to 25 per cent. No synergistic hypnotic effects were obtained in the dog (see page 206).

Numerous attempts have been made to interpret the specific cortical action of marihuana from the behavior of animals, particularly of dogs. In our observation, there is no conclusive indication of psychic alterations in dogs from any dose and still less in cats, rabbits or mice. The behavior of the dog is altered, but this can be explained as a consequence of the motor effects of marihuana rather than as a sign of not otherwise demonstrable psychic anomalies. The ataxia causes it to compensate for the motor and postural disturbance, and this affects its attention and reaction to external and internal stimuli. The rhesus monkey also failed to show psychic anomalies in some incidental experiments with doses producing a marked ataxia. Psychic alterations, if they exist, may become accessible to study by the methods of experimental psychology, especially by the use of higher primates.

Site of the Marihuana Action in Animals

The attempt to trace the effects of marihuana to the site of action leads to two somewhat paradoxical conclusions: (1) All the chief actions of marihuana—vomiting, scratching, as well as corneal areflexia and ataxia—are to be ascribed to a central nervous influence of the drug. Walton's remark, "Very few drugs are so limited to effects on the cerebral cortex and so lacking in peripheral effects[65]," is justified, if, by extending "cerebral cortex" to "brain," our lack of knowledge on the exact sites of attack within the brain is admitted. (2) Ataxia is the most important symptom of central nervous action, whereas the most prominent central sensory action, the "pleasure" action in man, is not observable in laboratory animals. It is tempting to assume that the ataxia is of cortical origin as is the production of euphoria in man. Some features common to both actions—the individual variation, the disturbing influence of stimuli, the apparent concomitance of both effects in man—may indicate closely related sites of action. On the other hand, a type of motor ataxia very similar to marihuana ataxia originates from anomalies at sites other than the cortex, namely, various parts of the paleoencephalon.

IV. The Approaches to the Discovery of the Active Principles of Marihuana

A. The Chemical Approach: Chemistry of the Class of Cannabinols.

It has long been known that the active principles of marihuana are practically insoluble in water and readily soluble in a variety of organic solvents, and are contained in the resinous or oily residue from alcohol, ether, acetone, benzene or petroleum ether extracts. Distillation of these residues under reduced pressure affords a crude preliminary method of concentrating the active principle.

From the first serious attempts to isolate the substances responsible for the specific action of hemp in 1896,[69] the crude distillate oil from organic extracts has been used as a starting material. No crystalline material was ever obtained from these oils, but fractional redistillation of hemp oil yielded a rather reproducible fraction, characterized by a relatively narrow range of boiling point. It could be further purified by fractional distillation, particularly when previously subjected to esterification. These oils had an almost uniform elementary composition, both before and after saponification. The product, of varying purity, resulting from these processes was called "cannabinol" and in its purest state the elementary formula was given as C_{20} or $_{21}$, H_{26} to $_{30}$, O_2. The cannabinol fraction amounted to a varying percentage of the redistillated oil; it appears highest in Oriental hemps.

Cannabinol

The discovery of cannabinol as a more or less pure chemical unit dates back as early as 1899. In that year a crystalline acetyl derivative was obtained from cannabinol fractions, and cannabinol recovered therefrom by hydrolysis (Wood et al.,[70] confirmed by Fraenkel[33]). For a long period all attempts at chemical identification were concentrated upon this cannabinol. For more than three decades, slow progress was made by various chemists in their efforts to discover the details of the chemical structure of cannabinol, culminating in R. S. Cahn's work in England. Cahn[29, 30] came very close to demonstrating the correct structural formula of cannabinol. He succeeded in 1932 (see Table 46, formula I) in demonstrating that the skeleton of cannabinol is a diphenyl, the two rings of which are also connected by an oxygen-containing bridge so that an interjacent pyran ring is formed, that one of the two rings carries an aromatic hydroxyl group and that there are four aliphatic side chains, three methyls and an *n*-amyl.

Only the positions of the amyl and the hydroxyl group at ring B were found to differ from Cahn's description, when the complete chemical configuration of cannabinol (II)*—isolated from American hemp — as 1-hydroxy-3-*n*-amyl-6,6,9-trimethyl-6-dibenzopyran ($C_{21}H_{26}O_2$) was demonstrated in 1939 by Adams and his collaborators. This they confirmed by synthesis of the crystalline substance of melting point 76-77° (corr.).[6] That the cannabinols from Indian and Egyptian hemp are identical with those reported by Adams, was shown in 1940 in Todd's Laboratory.[34, 36, 43]

CANNABIDIOL

About the same time, Adams et al. succeeded in isolating and fully identifying another crystalline component of the distillate oils, $C_{21}H_{30}O_2$, m.p. 66-67° (corr.), $[\alpha]^{27}$ −125°, which he called cannabidiol.[2, 3, 4, 5, 6] Its structure (III) showed a rather close relationship to cannabinol. It differs from cannabinol mainly in the lack of the third (pyran) ring. Instead, there is a second aromatic hydroxyl group at ring B and an isopropenyl group at ring A. In addition, one of the two carbon rings (A) of cannabidiol is partially reduced by the introduction of four hydrogens (the natural *l*-cannabidiol is 1, 2, 5, 6-tetrahydrogenated; Adams et al.[19]).

Cannabidiol was shown by Adams and his associates to give a very strong alkaline Beam test, as demonstrated by Cahn[30] for diols of this class. None of the other pure substances dealt with in this report

*All structural formulas (Roman numerals in text) are given in Table 46.

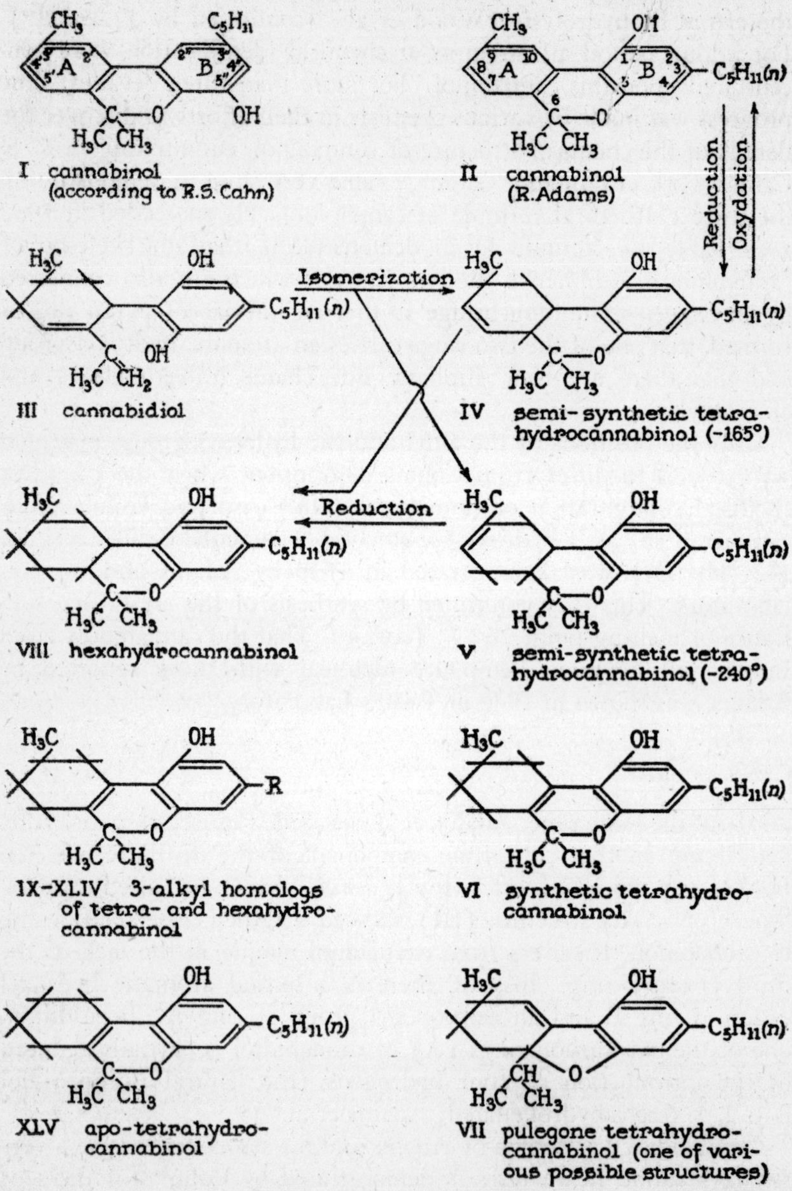

I cannabinol (according to R.S. Cahn)

II cannabinol (R.Adams)

Reduction / Oxydation

III cannabidiol

Isomerization

IV semi-synthetic tetrahydrocannabinol (−165°)

Reduction

VIII hexahydrocannabinol

V semi-synthetic tetrahydrocannabinol (−240°)

IX–XLIV 3-alkyl homologs of tetra- and hexahydrocannabinol

VI synthetic tetrahydrocannabinol

XLV apo-tetrahydrocannabinol

VII pulegone tetrahydrocannabinol (one of various possible structures)

TABLE 46.—Structure of Cannabinols and Related Substances. R, in IX-XLIV, stands for H or any *n*-alkyl from CH_3 to C_9H_{19}.

TABLE 46.—Continued.

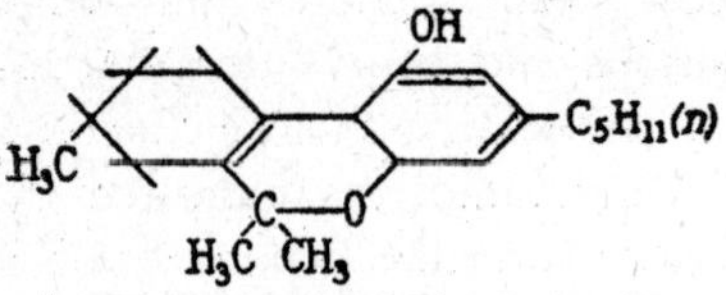

XLVI 8-methyl isomer of tetrahydrocannabinol

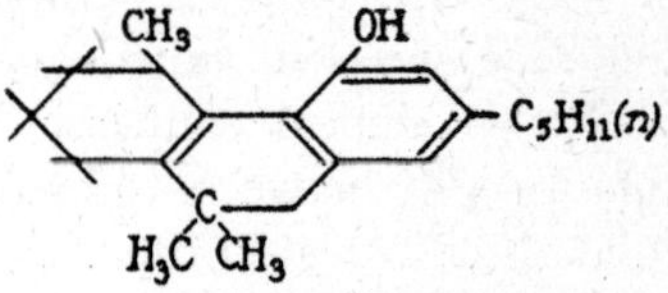

XLVII 10-methyl isomer of tetrahydrocannabinol

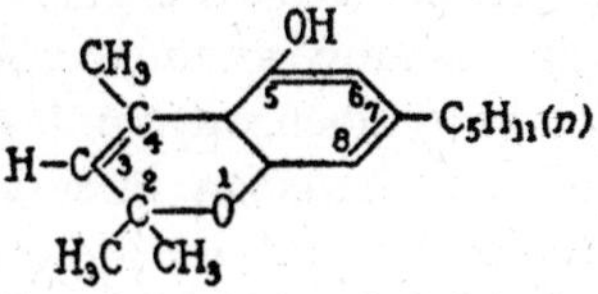

XLVIII 2,2,4-trimethyl-5-hydroxy-7-*n*-amyl-1,2-benzopyran

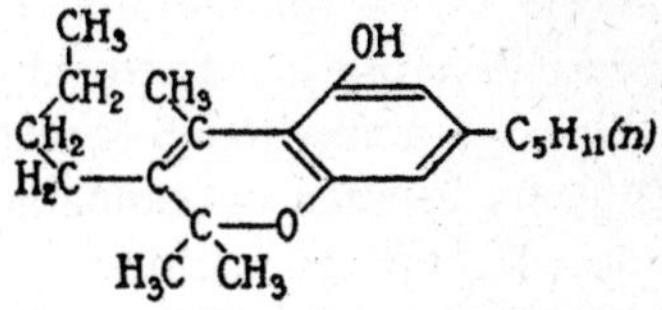

XLIX 2,2,4-trimethyl-5-hydroxy-3-*n*-butyl-7-*n*-amyl-1,2-benzopyran

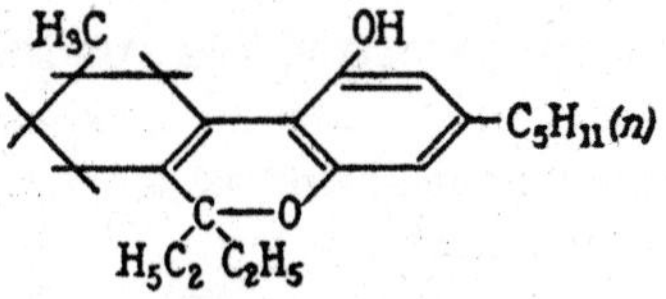

L 1-hydroxy-3-*n*-amyl-6,6-diethyl-9-methyl-7,8,9,10-tetrahydro-6-benzopyran

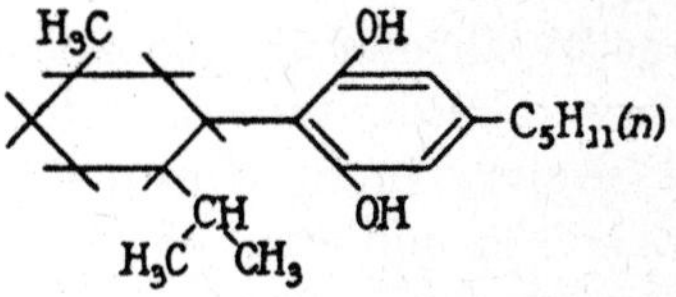

LI tetrahydrocannabidiol

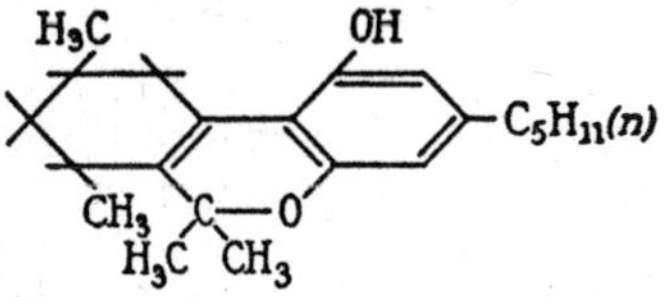

LII 7-methyl-tetrahydrocannabinol

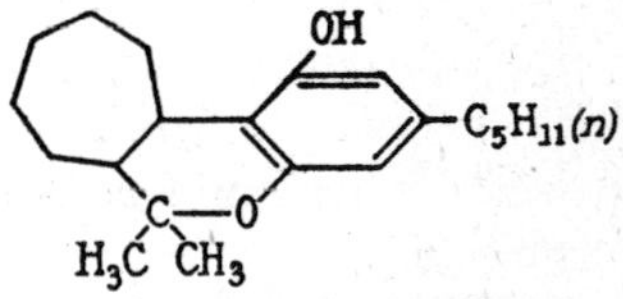

LIII cycloheptyl analog of tetrahydrocannabinol

was found to be Beam-positive. The Beam test exhibited by cannabidiol differs, however, from that of purified red oil. The color is more intense and deeper violet, whereas that from red oil is reddish violet. Therefore, the color given by red oil is obviously "dependent in part on substances other than cannabidiol" (Adams[2]).*

*The only other hemp components reactive in the alkaline Beam test are those of Fulton's[77] "IRAB" fraction; they differ from cannabidiol by being soluble in aqueous alkali, and were demonstrated in Todd's Laboratory[80] to be phenolic acid esters of cannabidiol.

TETRAHYDROCANNABINOL

Thus, two pure crystalline substances were isolated from hemp oils in a series of ingenious investigations and fully elucidated by brilliant chemical synthesis. In view of the relatively close chemical relationship between cannabinol and cannabidiol, as indicated by their structure and origin, it is tempting to form the hypothesis of a genetic relationship between the two. Both from cannabinol (II) (by reductive removal of two double bonds in A), and still more readily from cannabidiol (III) (by intramolecular isomerization through closing of the pyran ring), tetrahydrocannabinol (1-hydroxy-3-*n*-amyl-6,6,9-trimethyl-tetrahydro-6-dibenzopyran, $C_{21}H_{30}O_2$), an isomer of cannabidiol, should result as an intermediate product between cannabinol and cannabidiol, and its presence in marihuana oil is not improbable.

The isolation and to a greater extent the identification of a natural tetrahydrocannabinol from hemp oils was hampered by the fact that the tetrahydrocannabinols have no tendency to crystallize, to form crystalline derivatives, or to exhibit characteristic identity reactions. Therefore, proof of its homogeneity as a chemical unit is dependent upon the fulfilment of a number of other criteria:

1) Constancy in elementary composition
2) Constancy of boiling point
3) Typical specific rotation
4) Constant refractory index
5) Inability to further partition the material by means which have proven efficient in separating it from mixtures with closely related substances.[68]
6) Qualitatively and quantitatively typical biological effectiveness is one more important criterion to be added to the five listed above which were set up by Wollner and collaborators in case of a biologically active product.

It is on the basis of such proof that a number of substances having the structure of tetrahydrocannabinols have been isolated from hemp oil.

(1) One of these natural tetrahydrocannabinols, "charas tetrahydrocannabinol," was isolated and identified by the Narcotics Laboratory from an Oriental cannabis resin, charas, in the form of its acetate, $[\alpha]^{21}$ –214°, after hydrolysis $[\alpha]^{21}$–216°.[68]

(2) Another tetrahydrocannabinol was prepared earlier by the

same investigators from American hemp oil. This was separated in the nonadsorbable portion during passage of the pentane solution of a highly pre-purified acetylated oil fraction over an alumina column subsequent to removal of cannabidiol by oxidation. It is believed that this may represent the first natural tetrahydrocannabinol directly isolated from the plant source. The specific rotation of this acetate was –143°. Looking back, it now appears that, according to the above criteria, the same investigators (Wollner, Matchett and Loewe) had even earlier (1937) succeeded in isolating tetrahydrocannabinols from the natural source.

Two other tetrahydrocannabinols were obtained on an entirely different basis. In order to demonstrate the genetic relationship between cannabinol and cannabidiol and to find out how easily tetrahydrocannabinols can be formed from known components of hemp oil, Adams et al. studied the process of isomerization of cannabidiol *in vitro* and succeeded not only in preparing two "semi-synthetic" tetrahydrocannabinols from their pure crystalline cannabidiol by the aid of various condensing agents, but also in showing that the product varies in nature according to the choice of the method of condensing:[12, 13, 19]

(3) Tetrahydrocannabinol of the specific rotation $[\alpha]^{27}$ –130° (IV)*

(4) Tetrahydrocannabinol of the specific rotation $[\alpha]^{27}$ –265° (V)*

Their acetates had the rotation $[\alpha]^{34}$ –167° and $[\alpha]^{34}$ –229°, respectively, their methyl ethers $[\alpha]^{32}$ –166° and $[\alpha]^{32}$ –226°, respectively.

In a series of particularly interesting syntheses Adams et al. were able to prepare five completely synthetic tetrahydrocannabinols from starting materials of relatively simple structure:

(5) Racemic "synthetic" (7,8,9,10-) tetrahydrocannabinol (VI), resulting from condensing ethyl-5-methylcyclohexanone-2-carboxylate (to build ring A) and olivetol (to form ring B).[14]

(6) Racemic "pulegone tetrahydrocannabinol" (VII), obtained by condensing pulegone and olivetol.[16]

(7) An optically active, "synthetic," *d*-(7,8,9,10-) tetrahydrocannabinol, specific rotation $[\alpha]^{27}$ +152° (VIa[73]).

---

*Earlier products [12, 13] showed rotations of –160±10° and –225 to 240°, respectively; they were later considered[19] as mixtures of IV and VI.

(8) An optically active, "synthetic," *l*-tetrahydrocannabinol, specific rotation $[\alpha]^{27}$ −114° (VIb[78]).

(9) Another "synthetic" *l*-tetrahydrocannabinol having distinctly different physical criteria and different biological activity (VIc, unpublished).

Isomerism of Tetrahydrocannabinol

Cannabinol has numerous isomers, varying in the position of the alkyl and hydroxyl groups at the two aryl rings. In the case of cannabidiol, there exist two additional sources of isomerism, optical activity and variations in the position of the two double bonds. The same sources of isomerism exist in the case of tetrahydrocannabinol. The 1-hydroxy-3-*n*-amyl-6,6,9-methyl compound alone has a great number of isomers according to the position of the double bond. They represent four significantly different types, namely, (1) those with the double bond conjugated with the aromatic ring B (in 11,12 position), which have one asymmetric C-atom, position 9, (2) those in which the double bond includes the methyl-substituted C-atom 9 (8,9 or 9,10), which have two asymmetric C-atoms, 11 and 12, (3) those with the double bond touching the pyran ring (10,11 or 7,12), which have two asymmetric C-atoms, 9 and 10 or 9 and 12, and (4) those with the double bond touching neither the pyran ring nor C-atom 9 (7,8), which have 3 asymmetric C-atoms, in 9,11 and 12. Type 1 represents pyrans, all the others are really dihydropyran derivatives. Fundamentally there are two isomers of type 1, sixteen of types 2 and 3, namely four each in each of the four sub-groups, and eight isomers of type 4.

With respect to the semi-synthetic tetrahydrocannabinols, Adams has demonstrated that the representative with lower specific rotation is likely to have the double bond closer to the conjugated position than that exhibiting a higher rotation. He[11, 15, 73] assigned to the double bond of the former the 7,8 position, to that of the latter the 8,9 position, whereas the fully synthetic tetrahydrocannabinol (VI) has the double bond in conjugated position. Accordingly, these three substances should be representatives of type 4, type 2 and type 1, respectively. The exact position of the double bonds in the different natural tetrahydrocannabinols, which may or may not be the only characteristic distinguishing them from each other and from the semi-synthetic and synthetic isomers, is still an open question.

The double purpose of further elucidating the structural formulas and of studying the structure-activity relationship in this group of isomers gave origin to the synthesis of another series of isomers of tetrahydrocannabinol, namely, those differing in the position of the methyl group in ring A. In all the above-mentioned tetrahydrocannabinols, the methyl group is in a position meta to the linkage with the benzene ring B. Two isomers were synthesized by Adams and collaborators[17] with the methyl group in the positions para and ortho, respectively: 1) 6,6,8- (XLVI, m.p. 72-73°) and 2) 6,6,10-trimethyl-1-hydroxy-3-*n*-amyl-7,8,9,10-tetrahydro-6-dibenzopyran [XLVII, b.p. 181-185° (0.5-1.0 mm.)].

Isomers varying in the position of the phenolic hydroxyl group have been prepared in Todd's laboratory.[58a]

Other Reduction Products of Cannabinol

Tetrahydrocannabinol is a reduction product of cannabinol. Whereas the intermediate dihydrocannabinols have not been obtained, the end products with a completely hydrogenated ring A, the hexahydrocannabinols, $C_{21} H_{32} O_2$, have been prepared by Adams, both by reduction of cannabinol and tetrahydrocannabinols and by synthesis. The reduction products of the optically active semi-synthetic tetrahydrocannabinols are identical. This hexahydrocannabinol (VIII) has an optical rotation of $[\alpha]^{27}$ –70°.[18] In addition, two synthetic hexahydrocannabinols were prepared by Adams by the reduction of "synthetic tetrahydrocannabinol" and of pulegone tetrahydrocannabinol; both are optically inactive.[15]

Homologs of Tetrahydrocannabinol

A number of isomers of tetrahydrocannabinol were synthesized, as mentioned above, for the purpose of studying the significance of the position of the methyl side chain at ring A. Likewise a number of homologs were synthesized at the University of Illinois also for the purpose of studying the significance of variations in the side chains.

With regard to the 9-methyl in ring A, a homolog was synthesized in which this methyl group is missing (1-hydroxy-3-*n*-amyl-6,6-dimethyl-7,8,9,10-tetrahydro-6-dibenzopyran, apo-tetrahydrocannabinol, XLV[17]), another one with a 9-ethyl group (Adams et al., unpublished), and three with an additional methyl group, namely 6,6, 7,9-(LII),6,6,8,9-, and 6,6,9,9-tetramethyl-1-hydroxy-3-*n*-amyl-7,8,9, 10-tetrahydro-6-dibenzopyran (Adams et al., unpublished).

With respect to the two 6,6-methyl groups in the pyran ring, a homolog was synthesized with two ethyl (L), another with two *n*-propyl groups in the same position (Adams et al.),[17] and later a 6,6-di-*n*-butyl homolog (Bembry and Powell[24]).

A great variety of homologs was prepared by varying the length of the 3-alkyl chain in ring B. The number of such homologs was increased by using either one of the two synthetic tetrahydrocannabinols as a basis for these variations and also either one of the two reduction products. In this way, there were prepared:[16, 20] "synthetic tetrahydrocannabinol" homologs with a 3-alkyl chain of methyl, *n*-propyl,*n*-butyl,*n*-hexyl,*n*-heptyl and *n*-octyl (also: *iso*-amyl and *iso*-butyl, Russell et al.[58b]); the same six homologs of "synthetic hexahydrocannabinol"; six homologs of the "pulegone tetrahydrocannabinol" with a *n*-propyl,*n*-butyl,*n*-hexyl,*n*-heptyl,*n*-octyl and *n*-nonyl side chain in position 3; five homologs—3-*n*-propyl, 3-*n*-butyl, 3-*n*-hexyl, 3-*n*-heptyl and 3-*n*-octyl—of pulegone hexahydrocannabinol (IX-XLIV).

A homolog lacking the 1-hydroxyl group was also synthesized.[58b, 24]

Reduction Products of Cannabidiol

Cannabidiol also contains two double bonds available for reduction. A tetrahydrocannabidiol, in which the double bond in the cyclohexan ring A was removed and the isopropenyl group transformed into an isopropyl group, was prepared by Adams et al. (LI, unpublished).

Analogs of Tetrahydrocannabinol

In addition to these variations in the positions of double bonds and in the position and length of the various side chains, as well as in the presence or absence of the pyran ring, a series of other variations in the structure in this class of cannabinols was studied by opening ring A. This leads to a group of benzopyrans with no second carbon ring to the left. A benzopyran analog of tetrahydrocannabinol was thus synthesized with only a methyl group left in the place of ring A (2,2,4-trimethyl-5-hydroxy-7-*n*-amyl-1,2-benzopyran, XLVIII[18]). Another benzopyran was synthesized, having an open methyl and an open butyl group, i.e., an undiminished number of carbon atoms in aliphatic groupings, in the place of ring A (2,2,4-trimethyl-3-*n*-butyl-5-hydroxy-7-*n*-amyl-1,2-benzopyran, XLIX[18]). A third benzopyran was synthesized having cycloheptan in the place of ring A of tetrahydrocannabinol (LIII, unpublished).

Terpenes*)

A significant contribution to the knowledge of the components of hemp was made in 1942. In studying the lighter fractions of oils from Egyptian hemp, Simonsen and Todd[82] succeeded in identifying p-cymene and 1-methyl-4-isopropyl-benzene as the main components of a low-boiling, and humulene (α-caryophyllene), a component of hop and clove oils, in a higher-boiling terpene fraction. Obviously this group of hemp components contains materials available for the synthesis of cannabinols in the hemp plant.

Quebrachitol

For several reasons a chemical of entirely different structure may be included at the end of this chapter which is otherwise concerned with an enumeration of representatives of the cannabinol class. It completes the list of the chemically pure and structurally identified components of hemp. It is contained in the petrol ether solutions of crude red oil along with the cannabinols, and is separated by subjecting red oil to vacuum distillation, when it deposits high up in the fractionation column. It was isolated by Adams in the course of the investigations on the cannabinol class.[6]

This component of hemp oil is quebrachitol, $C_7 H_{14} O_6$, m.p. 192-193°, a monomethyl ether of the hexahydroxy-cyclohexane, *l*-inositol.

Genetic Relationship in the Cannabinol Class

Our knowledge of the chemistry of marihuana as here described has been reached in the span of a few years. Some of the various substances included and numerous others have been synthesized by the Illinois group of chemists for purposes of analyzing problems of chemical structure, but mention is made only of substances employed

*This section was inserted after the closing of the original report.

in connection with pharmacological problems. The achievements of the chemist have opened the approach to a new class of organic chemicals with a large number of representatives, which, although comprising certain di-phenol and benzopyran derivatives in addition to dibenzopyran derivatives, may be appropriately called the cannabinol class. The enormous gain in chemical knowledge can best be appreciated by comparing the host of substances described and analyzed since 1939 with the small number of compounds mentioned in Blatt's exhaustive survey of the chemistry of marihuana in 1938.[25]

This large family of new compounds embraces an impressive number of components of the hemp oils, in addition to a still greater number of new synthetic substances of the cannabinol class. To the biologist falls the responsibility of determining which, if any, of the natural products in this new class are responsible for the biological actions of the hemp preparations. The following chapters reveal the extent to which the isolation of the active principles was dependent upon the capacity of pharmacology to make available the techniques for a systematic approach to the problem.

In connection with the problem of the naturally occurring active principles, it is important to keep in mind that two pivotal points in the chemistry of the entire group are cannabinol and cannabidiol. It is apparent that cannabidiol is destined to be the starting material in a series of transformations which end in the formation of a much more stable product, cannabinol. This may explain the rather curious analytical data on hemp oils of different origin: Cannabidiol, which accounts for a high percentage of the oil from American hemp, is found in the oil from Oriental hashish only in small and irregular amounts. On the other hand, American hemp oil is poor in, or even devoid of cannabinol which in turn makes up a large portion of the oil from Oriental hemps. The genetic relationship is indicated by the observation that American hemp oil may also be poor in cannabidiol when prepared from older lots of hemp, particularly from herbs which have been subjected to years of withering on the stack. The crucial experiment has to our knowledge not been performed, namely, the examination of the cannabidiol content in extracts from freshly harvested Oriental herbs. At any rate, there is reason to believe that the tetrahydrocannabinols, among other representatives of the class, are intermediate products in the conversion of cannabidiol into cannabinol.

B. The Pharmacological Approach: Procedures for Quantitative Evaluation of Marihuana Actions.

Tests and Assays

The pharmacologist's rôle in the search of the unknown active principles is to identify them among the numerous fractionated and isolated products. This requires the application of pharmacological methods, the only characteristic of the unknown substances being their biological activity.

The pharmacological actions of marihuana suggest a number of biological tests. Such qualitative identity reactions serve to indicate the presence of active substances and are an essential aid to their isolation. Their usefulness in the problem of the purification of the unknown principles depends upon their specificity.

Even a specific qualitative test, however, may be a group reaction, characteristic of a multiplicity of agents of the same pharmacological class. Moreover, the steps of chemical fractionation may not always sharply separate effective from ineffective fractions. For both reasons, procedures for determining quantitatively the potencies of crude preparations and purified products are required in addition to qualitative reactions.

A test may be specific, but not convertible into a quantitative assay method, and vice versa. The measurement of potency involves two different steps, namely, (1) the creation of a yardstick, that is, of tools and standards for recording doses in terms of effect, and (2) the means for interpretation of the recorded observations in terms of the potency of the test material with reference to a standard material. A reliable yardstick requires that the effect vary in intensity to a measurable degree with the dosage and that this functional relationship of $\frac{\delta\ (\text{effect})}{\delta\ (\text{dose})}$ be known for at least a definite range of effect. The crucial criterion of the usefulness of a bioassay method is the reproducibility of the potency values obtained. Reproducibility requires knowledge of the inter- and intra-individual variations. It is with regard to these two requirements that the principles of interpretation must be developed.

Bioassay by Approximation

Almost all the test reactions for marihuana—the lethal action, general paralyzing actions, the corneal anesthesia, the ataxia, and the synergistic sleep-prolonging action—have been suggested for bioassay; only the latter three hold promise of specificity. The majority of the other actions can be dismissed from consideration.

To make tests useful in the chemical and pharmacological identification of active principles, it was necessary to adapt them to the requirements already mentioned. Before discussing the specific tests, an explanation of our general procedure for obtaining reliable potency values will be presented, since this was of decisive influence in the accurate evaluation of marihuana activity. The method was developed for similar purposes[45, 46, 48] and introduced in marihuana assays to overcome the difficulties of inter- and intra-individual variation as well as those caused by unfavorable trends in the dose-effect curve. Its principle is that of "approximation," since it establishes the potency value, which is the ratio between equi-effective doses of the standard and the test substance, by comparing doses of unequal effect rather than relying upon apparently equi-effective doses of test and standard substance. The greater conclusiveness of this procedure is due to the fact that it avoids conclusions made from an inconclusive range of dosage and that it reveals immediately, without further steps, the limits of accuracy of the individual assay in terms of the range of variation. The procedure is indispensable when the inter-individual variation in sensitivity is large, and expensive animals, or animals hard to handle in large numbers, have to be employed, as is the case in anesthesia tests in rabbits and ataxia tests in dogs.

Assay of Paralyzing Actions—the Goldfish Test

In the description of its author[56] the goldfish test is not a bioassay method. It is lacking in that a calibration of the toxicity of varied doses of the same preparation was not made. Single goldfish varying in weight from 3 to 5 Gm. were kept in individual basins containing 1,000 cc. water. Acetone extracts from different hemps were added in amounts such that every dose was equivalent to the same amount of dry herb, and the differences in potency were expressed by the differences in the time elapsing until death. Some of these extracts were assayed in the dog in our laboratory, and it can be seen (Table 49) that the differences between the goldfish "potencies" are qualitatively—but not quantitatively—similar to the ataxia potencies. Since further studies on this test are required to determine whether it can be used as an assay method for an essential marihuana principle, we made no use of it for identifying marihuana components.

Assay of Synergistic Hypnotic Action

The synergistic hypnotic action in the mouse[47] complies with the requirements for a yardstick. The duration of sleep is a function of the marihuana dose administered in combination with a constant basal dose of the hypnotic, pernoston. The inter-individual variation in sensitivity was considerable, but, as usual in the case of small and low-priced animals, it can be overcome by the use of sufficiently large single-dose groups (10-20 individuals). The intra-individual variation, which was marked even with reference to sensitivity to the basal hypnotic alone, was controlled by performing all the experiments with the test and the standard preparation on the same day. Even though large single-dose groups were employed, the method of approximation was helpful in finding potency values. It appears that even without extensive studies on reproducibility and without well-developed standards for routine use, the method is serviceable for identifying the synergistic hypnotic principle.

Assay in Rabbits

The corneal anesthesia test (Gayer Test)[38] in the rabbit is based upon a pharmacological phenomenon which has long been used for evaluating local anesthetics. The degree of corneal anesthesia is a function of the concentration of local anesthetic applied to the conjunctiva. The intensity of action is expressed by (1) the intensity of the anesthetic effect, (2) its duration, and (3) the extent of the anesthetized area. The intensity of effect is measured by counting the number of responses in a series of uniform applications of a calibrated hair to the cornea. The stimulus is applied to the central part of the cornea which is less susceptible to anesthetic action than the periphery. Walton[65, 66] obtained potency estimates for different preparations by recording positive responses in 20 trials at varying intervals after the intravenous administration of various doses. Whereas such procedures provide some information, neither Gayer nor others appear to have studied the inter- and intra-individual variability. That these variations are not negligible in the case of marihuana is indicated by incidental remarks of some of the authors.

In general, they determined relative potency by selecting doses giving equal responses. Figure 2 (also Figure 3, last example) gives examples of the poor reproducibility of such determination in our own experiments. The inter-individual variation is very marked. For instance, the doses of the standard (red oil) which elicited incomplete anesthesia (a 30 to 60 per cent response) in different animals vary about ±70 per cent from the mean, and doses with a 70 to 90 per cent response by about ±80 per cent. The intra-individual variation is still greater. The ratio between a weakly and a strongly effective dose of the standard (which should be <1.0) was variable—1.0, 2.0, 4.0 or 7.0; the ratio between the ataxia units of different preparations in doses of equal areflexia effectiveness was more than 78 in some instances. In most of the animals the susceptibility gradually

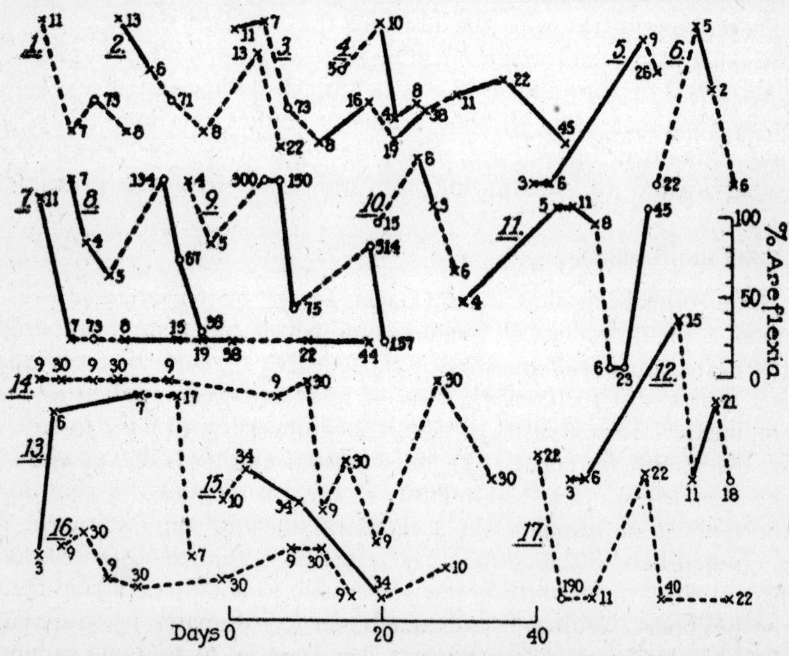

FIGURE 2.—Variations in the Corneal Areflexia Response to Marihuana. Ordinates: Degree of corneal areflexia—Abscissas: Duration of observation period. Curves represent the degrees of areflexia produced by successive doses of marihuana in each of 17 rabbits (No. 1 to 17). Figures at points on curves represent the dose of marihuana in units of ataxia potency. Broken lines connect doses of different preparations, straight lines, doses of the same preparation. o = pure tetrahydrocannabinols. x = impure preparations.

decreased over periods of weeks and months. This explains the ambiguous results which we obtained in applying the anesthesia method to crude and pure marihuana products.

Assay in Dogs

The ataxia action in the dog, which has the merit of specificity, has been used for assaying marihuana for more than half a century. Nevertheless, there is disagreement regarding its value. Some investigators report no relationship between dose and intensity of effect, and some emphasize the difficulty due to a large variation in susceptibility. On the other hand, the U. S. Pharmacopoeia accepted a bioassay procedure for the evaluation of officinal Cannabis preparations based upon the ataxia action in the dog (extensively in ed. IX, briefly in ed. X, dropped in ed. XI). The procedure in all bioassay methods employing the ataxia action has been to determine doses giving equal responses in a restricted number of dogs. Apparently, no attempt has been made to eliminate the inter-individual variability by large groups of single-dose experiments. Instead, it has been recommended that the comparison of test and standard dose be repeated in reverse order in the same animal. By this procedure, which makes the assay very time-consuming, bioassays were often considered satisfactory when performed on only two dogs.

In Table 47 are given some figures regarding these questions which were obtained in our own bioassay experiments involving about 1,800 tests. Animals used in this study were observed over varying periods of time up to thirty-three months. An interval of at least three days was allowed between each injection, the average number per animal being about 50, and the highest number 114. Twenty-seven per cent were calibration experiments.

The great inter-individual variation is indicated by a standard deviation of 2.38 from a mean $E.D._{50}$ of 3.65 ($= \pm 77$ per cent). The average intra-individual variation was computed by comparing the dose-response ($E.D._{50}$) in an initial period of observation with that in a later period in the same animal. In some animals, more than two observation periods could be analyzed due to the length of the total period. The mean value, 3.65, obtained in all these periods including both sexes, is practically the same as that obtained in the initial period, 3.44. This indicates that the average sensitivity

TABLE 47

Reproducibility of ataxia effect in the dog—Survey of calibration experiments

No. of animals	Sex	Observation period: months	Longest observation period in group: months	Shortest observation period in group: months	Highest total number of experiments in one animal	Lowest total number of experiments in one animal	Highest number of calibration experiments in one animal	Lowest number of calibration experiments in one animal	Average total number of experiments per animal	Average number of calibration experiments per animal	Highest sub-threshold dose in group: Mg./Kg.	E. D. 50	Lowest dose of IV effect in group	Highest E.D. 50 in one animal	Lowest E.D. 50 in one animal
15*	M	13.3	33	1	114	4	27	3	56.0	14.8	4.0	3.10	2.8		
14*	F	11.5	33	0.3	112	3	29	3	44.1	12.3	3.4	3.79	1.4		
29*	M&F	12.5	33	0.3	114	3	29	3	50.2	13.5	4.0	3.44	1.4		
11†	M	16.4	33	7	—	—	27	11	—	18.0	4.8	5.03	4.7		
8†	F	16.4	33	7	—	—	29	10	—	16.4	4.3	2.51	1.4		
19†	M&F	16.4	33	7	—	—	29	10	—	17.5	4.8	3.97	1.4		
—	M&F‡	—	33	0.3	—	—	29	3	—	—	4.8	3.65	1.4	11.0	0.95

*Initial period
†Later period.
‡All 48 observation periods.

M = 3.65
Std. Dev. = 2.38

of the subjects to marihuana did not undergo an appreciable change. Actually, the mean value of 3.97 for the later observation periods indicates an average decrease in sensitivity of only 15 per cent. The result is different in each sex, the males showing a decrease in sensitivity of 62 per cent, the females an increase of 34 per cent. A closer analysis of the results from individual animals showed that generally a change in susceptibility, particularly the decrease in males, originates from a different postural behavior in response to the early as compared to the later doses. Only those animals which learn to maintain the upright position by vigorous compensatory action, and so disguise the ataxia, show the decrease. This compensatory action is most effectively displayed by strong and tense males. The entire phenomenon of apparent hypersensitivity in an initial period is thus probably to be explained by better adaptation to the motor requirements of the ataxia in later periods. It is not surprising that, discounting the initial changes, a satisfactory relationship between dose and intensity of ataxia is manifested in numerous recalibration experiments. This is illustrated by some examples in Figure 3.

Intra-individual variability can thus be eliminated as an appreciable source of error, and in this respect the ataxia method is obviously superior to the corneal anesthesia method. The considerable inter-individual variability, however, indicates the desirability of making comparisons from experiments in one and the same individual only. The "approximation method" becomes a necessity if under such circumstances information on the potency is to be obtained. The accuracy of the comparison must be checked by means of calculations of the variability (see page 174). Some deviation is unavoidable in any bioassay method because of factors which limit the reproducibility of the method; in part it depends upon the number of experiments performed with the test substance and the perfection of previous calibration with the standard. The data in Tables 49 and 50 on our assays show that even with two or three animals the range of deviation may be less than ±15 per cent, and that with larger numbers the accuracy can be further improved to ±5 per cent or less. The entire assay can be performed in one day. This compares favorably with the best results reported by one of the most careful users of procedures previously available; it requires "about 6 trials, all with the same dog" (that is, eighteen days) to obtain "an estimated accuracy of 10 to 15 per cent." [65, 66]

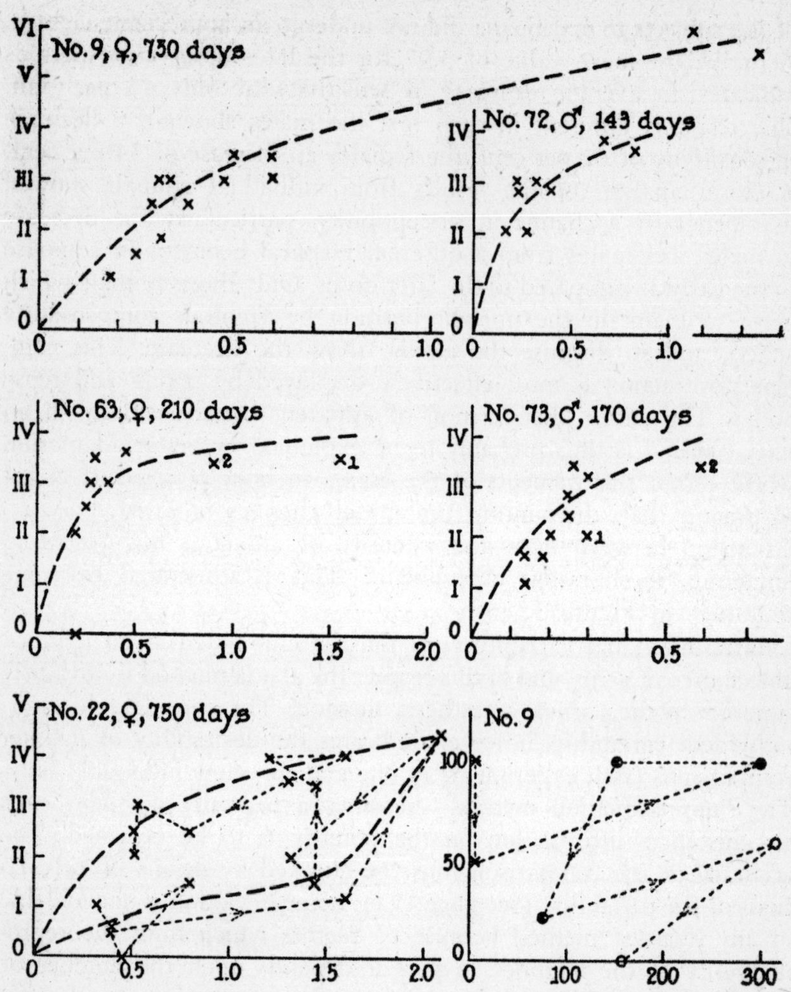

FIGURE 3.—Relationship between Dose and Intensity of Ataxia Effect. Individual curves are dose-action curves of ataxia in dogs No. 9, 22, 63, 72 and 73, and, for comparison, corneal areflexia in rabbit No. 9. Ordinate: Intensity of effect (expressed in grades of ataxia and in percentage areflexia respectively), Abscissa: dose (in dogs: in terms of mg./Kg. of standard preparation,—in rabbit: units of ataxia potency). In the case of dog 22 and rabbit 9 the time sequence of single experiments in the course of the total observation period is indicated by arrows.—Dog No. 22 was chosen as an example of the rare case in which the scatter was too wide to comply with a single smooth curve. Here, however, in contrast to the scatter in rabbit No. 9, the explanation is obvious: This female changed its sensitivity only at a certain time, after a number of pregnancies; the preceding and the subsequent halves of the total two-year observation period are represented by different smooth curves (broken lines).

Assay in Man

Evaluation in human test objects should be based upon the most specific test reaction which offers a direct approach to the euphoria-producing principle. A few experiments with Dr. E. Kahn made on ourselves (Modell and Loewe) with a natural tetrahydrocannabinol were adequate to demonstrate the wide inter-individual variation, the great influence of environmental and emotional factors upon the intensity of effect, that is, the existence of large intra-individual variations, and the enormous obstacles to the establishment of an objective standard for measuring the intensity of effect in humans.

* * *

In summary, our investigation of test and assay methods for the marihuana principles has resulted in making available a number of serviceable procedures. Some of them are improved methods for qualitative identification—such as the determination of the lethal dose, the production of corneal anesthesia, and the observation of alterations in pulse rate and blood pressure—which can be used either to determine which parts of the pharmacological action of the crude drug are associated with the chemical substances isolated, or to exclude such an association. The procedure based upon the synergistic hypnotic action in the mouse, although developed for quantitative purposes, must also, in its present state, be included among those more qualitative means of identification. This leaves the ataxia method as the best and only adequate representative of procedures which have been developed for quantitative purposes.

V. The Active Principles of Marihuana—Structure-Activity Relation In the Cannabinol Class

In our investigations on the active principles of marihuana, for technical reasons we have been guided by the ataxia effects in the dog. In addition, for almost 100 years (Liautaud, 1844[49]), the ataxia effect in the dog has been considered an experimental indicator of the cortical action in man, an assumption which has been sanctioned by the acceptance of the ataxia test in the U. S. Pharmacopoeia.

The potency of pure substances isolated from hemp oils was

TABLE 49

Ataxia potency of extracts and fractionation products of marihuana

No.	Preparation	Solids Gm. per 100 cc.	Potency (Reference to synthetic tetrahydro-cannabinol*)	Remarks	
				Interval to death in Robinson Goldfish Test min.	Dose p. liter bath fluid in equivalents of herb Gm.
	Extracts				
1	Commercial U.S.P. fluidextract (Brand A)	—	.061		
2	Roumanian No. 1	11.4	.033		
3	Manchurian No. 5	8.4	.019		
4	Italian No. 18	8.7	.014		
5	Tunisian	9.4	.520	68	0.2
6	Ferramington	8.1	.130	267	0.2
7	Manchurian No. 6	5.0	.060	1440	0.6
8	Kentucky No. 1	6.5	.087	1440	0.6
9	Kentucky No. 2	9.5	.048		
10	Kentucky No. 3	9.3	.048		
11	Illinois No. 42	8.0	.042		
12	Illinois No. 29	—	.087		
13	Illinois No. 7E	—	.043		
14	Minnesota No. E2	—	.021		
15	Minnesota No. E23	—	.028		
16	Minnesota No. E1F	—	.024		
17	Minnesota No. 38	—	.047		
18	Minnesota No. 39	33.1	.018		
19	Minnesota No. A Lot 3	23.1	.065		
20	Minnesota No. A Lot 7	33.6	.065		
21	Minnesota No. III, Lot 1	14.1	.130		

*cc. of extract referred to Gm. of standard.

TABLE 49—continued

No.	Preparation	Optical rotation	Potency (reference to synthetic tetrahydrocannabinol)	
			Mean	Range (±)
	Distilled Oils			
22	Red Oil No. 43 (from Extract No. 10)	—	.89	
23	Red Oil "Standard"	—	1.24	
24	Redistillate Red Oil "Standard"	—	4.33	
25	Purified Red Oil, Cannabidiol removed	—	6.80	
	Example of a Fractionated Redistillation (Acetates):			
26	Fraction 1	− 16.6	2.17	
27	Fraction 2	−137.7	3.25	
28	Fraction 3	−169.7	2.60	
29	Fraction 4	−170.4	2.68	
30	Fraction 5	−163.0	3.07	
31	Fraction 6	−158.6	2.17	
32	Fraction 7	−126.0	.54	
	Example of Distribution and Progressive Purification of Oriental Resin:			
33	Crude Distillate	−120.0	8.66	1.30
	Acetylated and passed over Silica Gel:			
34	Non-adsorbed from benzine	−180.0	6.71	.67
35	Adsorbed	—	1.00	.22
36	No. 34, non-adsorbed by activated alumina + "Hi Flo"; solvent: carbon tetrachloride	−195.0	6.54	.78
37	No. 34, non-adsorbed by same adsorbent; solvent: "Skelley-Solve"	−205.0	2.38	1.08
38	Same material as No. 35, redistilled, 4 peak fractions of equal potency; average	—	12.38	2.33
39	Combined 4 fractions, passed over "Alumina-Super Cal.", solvent: pentane; non-adsorbed	—	14.60	1.05
40	Eluate from above adsorbents with carbon tetrachloride	—	1.99	—
41	Hydrolysate of acetate No. 39 by acid	−216.0	8.01	1.73

measured by the ataxia activity and further studied in relation to the structural peculiarities of the cannabinols which appear to govern marihuana activity. All the steps of fractionation had to be checked with the aid of the ataxia method. A brief introductory review of the activity of preparations of varying purity will be given to illustrate the way they served in the isolation of the pure substances. Finally, the attempts to identify the hemp components responsible for other actions of the drug will be reviewed and it will be shown with the aid of potency indices how different products vary with regard to their relative potency in different test procedures.

All data on the activity of intermediate preparations and pure substances are expressed in terms of effectiveness relative to a standard substance. As our investigations progressed, the standard for ataxia potency had to be changed several times. Originally the findings were referred to a distillate red oil (Table 49, No. 23). Later on, a highly potent redistillate oil fraction (Table 49, No. 24) was chosen. However, when a pure synthetic substance, "synthetic tetrahydrocannabinol," became available, this compound was adopted as the standard of reference (Table 50, No. 16).* The factors of conversion from one standard to the other may be found in the following table:

TABLE 48

Factor of conversion of potency determined with reference to standard:	into potency with reference to:		
	Red Oil:	Pure Oil:	Synthetic Tetrahydrocannabinol:
Red Oil	1.00	0.29	1.24
Pure Oil	3.50	1.00	4.33
Synthetic Tetrahydrocannabinol	0.81	0.23	1.00

The potencies exhibited in actions other than ataxia were referred to other convenient standards. Potency indices, of course, were derived only from potencies referring to the same standard.

*At various times different standards have been used in previous publications, and in some instances the figures given there are, for this reason, at variance with those given in the present report.

Activity of Various Preparations of Marihuana

The ataxia potencies of a variety of impure marihuana preparations are assembled in Table 49. Some of the potency figures refer to products from successive steps in purification, others to extracts of varying origin tested in the search for a suitable source of material. The bulk of these were fluidextracts. In some instances, the solid content of these extracts is tabulated to give an idea of the yield in extractives. These figures also serve to indicate the variations in the amount of active principles in the resin. The assumption that such material has a constant potency is certainly not justified when Oriental hemps are compared with Occidental material, nor can the ratio between the components of lower and higher potency be considered constant in Occidental hemps.

Among the fluidextracts enumerated in Table 49 are three ("A Lot 3," "A Lot 7" and "III Lot 1") which were evaluated for use in the clinical experiments of the Mayor's Committee on Marihuana, and a commercial fluidextract A manufactured by an American pharmaceutical house. This extract, although several years old, was found to be of relatively high potency, did not deteriorate during the period of our work and was of greater potency than a solid extract B from another manufacturer.

The figures in Table 49 indicate a marked difference between the specimens of Oriental and American hemp examined. The extract from Oriental hemp, even though it was grown on American soil, had a higher potency. The difference is not explained by difference in the amounts of extractives. The same difference was found between the distillate oils; thus a charas distillate oil had twice the potency of a redistillate oil from Minnesota hemp.

American extracts from various sources also varied considerably in potency, namely, between 0.0034 and 0.087, as compared with a potency of 0.061 for the commercial U.S.P. fluidextract A.

The lowest value was found in an herb—but only one out of various harvests—grown under experimental conditions (Arlington Field of the Department of Agriculture). The low potency in this case is of particular interest, since the yield in extractives was high. Material which had been stacked outdoors had greater potency.

The data on redistillate oils show that the active substances can be concentrated in certain distillate fractions, but cannot be purified further by additional distillations or sharper fractionation. Such procedures result only in additional fractions of approximately the same potency (see Table 49, No. 25-30).

The example of an entire fractionation (No. 33-40, Table 49) illustrates particularly well the point that the effectiveness of purification by fractionated high-vacuum distillation falls short of the final goal. The refined process of molecular distillation introduced into the field of marihuana investigations by the Washington chemists leads somewhat closer. But it was through additional purification by selective adsorption of impurities that the final isolation of the active principle was achieved. This procedure was first applied to hashish by Bergel and Todd.[23, 71] It was, however, only by the combination of several expedients that the Washington investigators succeeded in isolating pure active principles. These expedients were: acetylation of the highly purified oils before subjecting them to adsorption in the Tswett column, careful choice of the adsorbents as well as the solvents, and repeated adsorption with variations of adsorbents and solvents.

The Active Principles of Marihuana and Their Potency

Ataxia Activity

Table 50 presents data on the ataxia potency of pure substances isolated from marihuana. Roman numerals in the last column refer to the structural formula in Table 46. Neither cannabidiol, the substance of greatest chemical lability and, accordingly, the starting material in the supposed chain of chemical transformations in the marihuana oils, nor cannabinol, the end-product of these natural alterations, was found to produce ataxia. Intermediate substances in the cannabidiol → cannabinol conversion were discovered to be the representatives of marihuana activity: The various tetrahydrocannabinols isolated from marihuana were all potent.

The greatest potency is respresented by the charas tetrahydrocannabinol isolated by the Washington investigators. Its acetate has a potency of 14.6, and the free alcohol, the form in which the substance exists in the natural product, can be assumed to be somewhat more potent (see page 204). The marihuana tetrahydrocannabinol (acetate) of the same investigators has a potency of 10.8. This means that the active principle has at least from 230 to 500 times the potency of the dried herb, and that the herb contains less than from

0.20 to 0.43 per cent of active principle of such outstanding potency. Another group of natural marihuana tetrahydrocannabinols varies in potency between 7.4 and 9.3. The optical rotation indicates that this group represents at least two different tetrahydrocannabinols. Further investigation will determine whether they are identical with the two semi-synthetic tetrahydrocannabinols prepared by Adams. If they should turn out to be the only active principles in the original crude extract, they would constitute a slightly higher percentage of the herb, namely, about 0.28 to 0.62 per cent.*

The assumption that the genetic relationship between the three main representatives of the cannabinol group in hemp oil is of the nature of cannabidiol → tetrahydrocannabinal → cannabinol, or at least that tetrahydrocannabinol is formed from cannabidiol by influences which act upon the plant or its excretion product under natural conditions, is now, since the pure substances have become available, supported by some experimental evidence. Ultraviolet light was studied as one of the possible natural influences. Our experiments in collaboration with the Narcotics Laboratory, Washington, D. C., had shown that ultraviolet irradiation does not appreciably diminish the ataxia potency of natural tetrahydrocannabinol. When, however, the ineffective crystalline cannabidiol was irradiated for twenty-four hours in an appropriate solvent by Dr. Adams in the Illinois laboratory, it gained an ataxia potency of 0.16. On the assumption that the active derivative formed through the influence of the radiant energy had a potency around 8.0, it appears that about 2 per cent of the cannabidiol was converted into tetrahydrocannabinol.

Synergistic Hypnotic Action

In a few experiments, summarized in Figure 4, pure natural compounds belonging to the cannabinol class have been studied with reference to the synergistic hypnotic action in the mouse. Neither pure cannabinol nor the semi-synthetic 8,9-tetrahydrocannabinol had a noticeable effect, whereas cannabidiol is markedly effective in doses

*The isolation of a substance from American hemp with a potency greater than the most active tetrahydrocannabinol from Oriental resin has been announced by Haagen-Smit in a preliminary communication.[40] Complete chemical data have not been presented, but it was a crystalline product and its method of preparation suggests an isomeric tetrahydrocannabinol. Its activity was tested on the dog and found to be very high, perhaps ten times that of even the most potent tetrahydrocannabinol thus far studied. Unfortunately the available quantity was sufficient for only two tests, so the evaluation of potency has but "very limited significance."[50]

TABLE 50

Current Number	Substance	Number of experiments	Potency (reference to synthetic tetrahydrocannabinol)		Structure
			Mean	Range (±)	
1	Cannabidiol, cryst.	10	<0.056		III
2	Cannabinol	8	Ineffective		II
3	Natural Tetrahydrocannabinol (Charas), Acetate, −214°	5	14.6	1.05	
4	Natural Tetrahydrocannabinol, less purified, −213.6°	10	13.0	1.30	
5	Natural Tetrahydrocannabinol, less purified, −212.6°	8	13.1	2.70	
6	Natural Tetrahydrocannabinol, acetate hydrolyzed by acid, −216°	7	8.0	1.73	
7	Natural Tetrahydrocannabinol acetate, dubious purity, −205°	11	6.5	0.78	
8	Natural Tetrahydrocannabinol (No. 7, hydrolyzed), −220°	15	7.8	0.47	
9	Natural Tetrahydrocannabinol, acetate	10	10.8	2.16	
10	Semi-synthetic Tetrahydrocannabinol, −165°	13	9.3	2.90	IV
11	Semi-synthetic Tetrahydrocannabinol, repurified, −160°	11	8.2	2.17	IV
12	Semi-synthetic Tetrahydrocannabinol, −130°	18	6.5	0.65	IV
13	Semi-synthetic Tetrahydrocannabinol, −260°	4	7.6	1.08	V
14	Semi-synthetic Tetrahydrocannabinol, −265°	20	7.3	0.89	V
15	Semi-synthetic Tetrahydrocannabinol, −260°	4	7.8	0.78	V
16	Synthetic Tetrahydrocannabinol, ± 0°	20	1.00	—	VI
17	Synthetic Tetrahydrocannabinol, + 152°	10	0.38	0.02	
18	Synthetic Tetrahydrocannabinol, −114°	9	1.66	0.21	
19	Synthetic Pulegone Tetrahydrocannabinol, −70°	11	0.58	0.12	VII
20	Dihydrocannabinol (Bergel et al., 22)	?	about 0.5 (estimated)		
21	Hexahydrocannabinol, synthetic, ± 0°	6	0.51	0.08	VIII
22	Hexahydrocannabinol, semi-synthetic, −70°	7	3.03	0.43	
23	Hexahydrocannabinol, pulegone	6	0.64	0.10	
24	Tetrahydrocannabidiol	4	<0.04		LI
	Other Benzopyrans				
25	Cycloheptyl analog (of Nr. 20): 3,4-cycloheptane-5-hydroxy-7-*n*-amyl-1,2-benzopyran	4	0.2	—	LIII

26	2,2,4-trimethyl-5-hydroxy-7-*n*-amyl-1,2-benzopyran	10	0.03	0.10	XLVIII
27	2,2,4-trimethyl-5-hydroxy-3-*n*-butyl-7-*n*-amyl-1,2-benzopyran	5	0.04	0.10	XLIX
	Esters and Ethers of Tetrahydrocannabinols				
28	Acetate of No. 10	—	about 1.04		
29	Acetate of No. 13	—	0.91	0.39	
30	Methyl ether of No. 10	—	<0.27		
31	Methyl ether of No. 13	—	<0.13		
	Synthetic Isomers and Homologs of Tetrahydrocannabinol *Alterations referring to Methyl Groups:*				
32	Minus 9-methyl: 1 hydroxy-3-*n*-amyl-6,6-dimethyl-7,8,9,10-tetrahydro-6-dibenzopyran	4	0.13	0.05	XLV
33	Methyl in position ortho: 1-hydroxy-3-*n*-amyl-6, 6,10-trimethyl-7,8,9,10-tetrahydro-6-dibenzopyran	6	0.25	0.05	XLVII
34	Methyl in position para: 1-hydroxy-3-*n*-amyl-6,6,8-trimethyl-7,8,9,10-tetrahydro-6-dibenzopyran	6	0.14	0.01	XLVI
35	Additional (7-)methyl: 1-hydroxy-3-*n*-amyl-6,6,7,9-tetramethyl-7,8,9,10-tetrahydro-6-dibenzopyran	10	0.75	0.08	LII
36	Additional (8-)methyl: 1-hydroxy-3-*n*-amyl-6,6,8,9-tetramethyl-7,8,9,10-tetrahydro-6-dibenzopyran	10	0.11	0.03	
37	Additional (9-)methyl: 1-hydroxy-3-*n*-amyl-6,6,9,9-tetramethyl-7,8,9,10-tetrahydro-6-dibenzopyran	7	0.10	0.02	
38	9-ethyl homolog	5	0.18	0.03	
39	6,6-diethyl homolog	8	0.12	0.02	L
40	6,6-di-*n*-propyl homolog	5	0.04	0.01	
	Alterations referring to n-amyl group: *Homologs of Synthetic Tetrahydrocannabinol*				
41	Methyl homolog	3	0.16	0.03	X
42	*n*-propyl homolog	2	0.40	0.08	XII
43	*n*-butyl homolog	4	0.38	0.13	XIII
[16	*n*-amyl homolog	20	1.00	—	VI]
44	*n*-hexyl homolog	7	1.82	0.40	XIV
45	*n*-heptyl homolog	10	1.05	0.15	XV
46	*n*-octyl homolog	7	0.66	0.13	XVI

TABLE 50—continued

Current Number	Substance	Number of experiments	Potency (reference to synthetic tetrahydrocannabinol)		Structure
			Mean	Range (±)	
	Homologs of Synthetic Hexahydrocannabinol				
47	—H homolog (no alkyl)	1	<0.10		XVIII
48	Methyl homolog	2	<0.04		XIX
49	*n*-propyl homolog	2	0.26	0.04	XXI
50	*n*-butyl homolog	3	0.37	0.06	XXII
[21	*n*-amyl homolog	6	0.51	0.08	VIII]
51	*n*-hexyl homolog	7	1.86	0.37	XXIII
52	*n*-heptyl homolog	10	0.83	0.18	XXIV
53	*n*-octyl homolog	4	0.24	0.06	XXV
	Homologs of Pulegone Tetrahydrocannabinol				
54	*n*-propyl homolog	3	<0.24		XXX
55	*n*-butyl homolog	4	0.25	0.10	XXXI
[19	*n*-amyl homolog	11	0.58	0.12	VII]
56	*n*-hexyl homolog	7	1.22	0.12	XXXII
57	*n*-heptyl homolog	9	1.15	0.15	XXXIII
58	*n*-octyl homolog	4	1.37	0.25	XXXIV
59	*n*-nonyl homolog	6	0.18	0.04	XXXV
	Homologs of Pulegone Hexahydrocannabinol				
60	*n*-propyl homolog	3	<0.20		XXXIX
61	*n*-butyl homolog	2	<0.15		XL
[23	*n*-amyl homolog	6	0.64	0.10	]
62	*n*-hexyl homolog	9	0.78	0.22	XLI
63	*n*-heptyl homolog	8	0.83	0.17	XLII
64	*n*-octyl homolog	5	<0.25		XLIII

between 10 and 20 mg./Kg. Compared with the effectiveness of American red oil in the same test, this figure indicates that the latter contained between 25 and 50 per cent of cannabidiol. This agrees with other evidence. An investigation of all natural tetrahydrocannabinols and other pure components would be necessary to prove that cannabidiol is the only representative of this action.

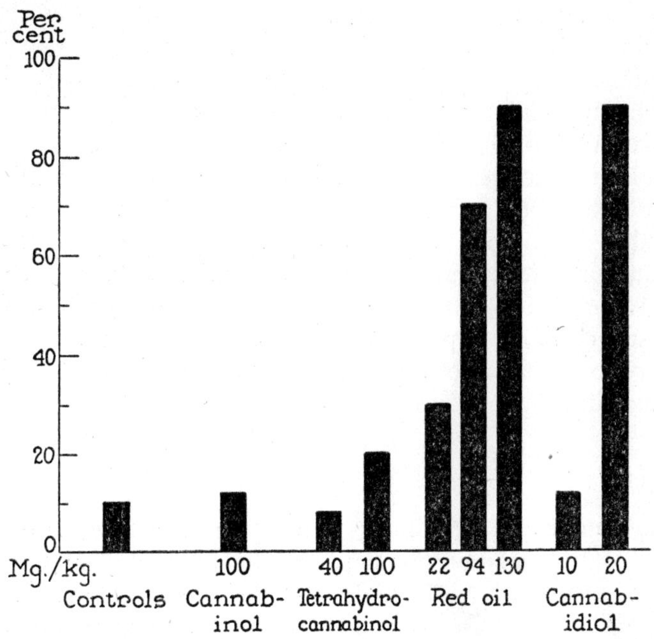

FIGURE 4.—Synergistic Hypnotic Action of Marihuana Components and a Barbiturate in the Mouse.

Ordinate: Percentage of animals in single-dose group in which the duration of sleep was over 100 minutes.

It is clear that the active principles responsible for the ataxia and for the synergistic hypnotic action are not the same. The synergistic hypnotic effect of cannabidiol is the biological equivalent of the chemical cannabidiol test (Beam test) that played such a large and unfortunately misleading rôle in the early period of marihuana research (see page 154).

Corneal Areflexia Action in the Rabbit

Cannabidiol and cannabinol did not produce corneal areflexia, but a number of tetrahydrocannabinols had considerable activity. Impure oil mixtures (red oil), however, were significantly more effective than the tetrahydrocannabinols.

The British group of investigators who confirmed the chemical findings of the Illinois group as well as our own findings on the specific activity, examined the latter solely through use of the areflexia action. They assumed that the areflexia action is specific for tetrahydrocannabinols and in all respects equivalent to the ataxia action, but they did not measure the potency indices of the ataxia and areflexia actions of their material, a step in our work which suggested that a third principle, not identical with those producing ataxia or synergistic hypnotic action, may be responsible for corneal areflexia. A possible explanation for their assumption may be found in the great intra-individual variation which we think makes the areflexia action valueless for assay purposes. Either the British investigators were satisfied by an approximate test procedure, or they developed a method of areflexia evaluation which eliminates the obstacles to reproducibility.*

Lethality

Some data from experiments with pure substances answer the question of the relationship between the fatal dose in the rabbit which is particularly susceptible and the specific actions in other species. A highly purified redistillate oil from marihuana (Table 49, No. 24; potency: 4.33) was lethal in doses varying between 2.3 and 8.4 mg./Kg. This agrees with the $L.D._{50}$ of 4 mg./Kg. reported by Bergel et al.[22] for their "Cannabinol fraction II." The $L.D._{50}$ of cannabidiol was 60 mg./Kg. in six intravenous experiments in the dog, that of semi-synthetic tetrahydrocannabinol (–160°) was between 32.5 and 43.2 mg./Kg., that of semi-synthetic tetrahydrocannabinol (-265°) was greater than 17 mg./Kg.

Obviously, neither cannabidiol nor tetrahydrocannabinol accounts for the high toxicity of crude preparations or the toxicity of impure or even repeatedly redistilled oils. The lethal action in the rabbit and the specific activity may therefore be due to different principles.

*The answer to this question will be found in the postscript on page 202.

Circulatory and Respiratory Actions

Electrocardiograms were obtained from a dog at the height of an ataxia-effective dose of charas tetrahydrocannabinol, but did not differ from control tracings.

A few experiments were conducted to determine the effect of marihuana on the pulse rate and to find out if it were caused by any of the pure principles. The results are demonstrated in the graph of a representative experiment in a well calibrated, non-narcotized dog (Figure 5).

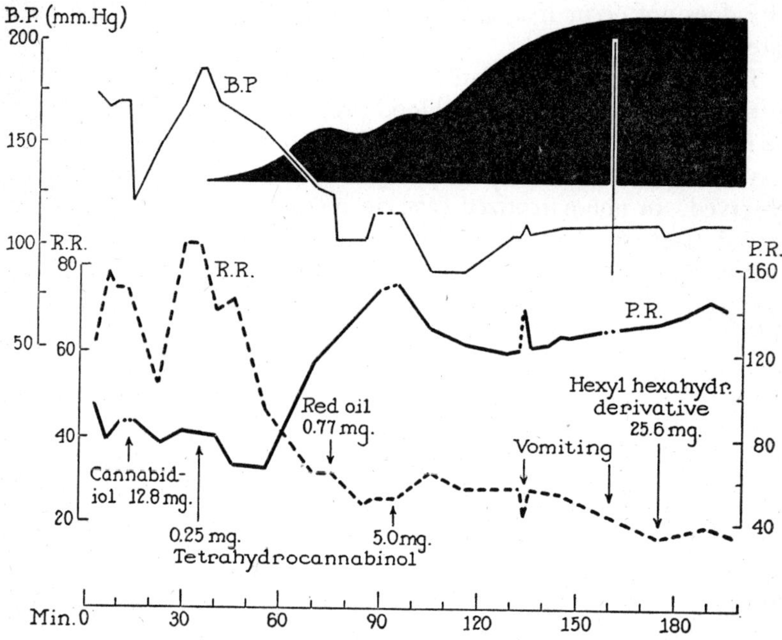

Figure 5.—Influence of Tetrahydrocannabinol upon Pulse Rate (P.R.) and Blood Pressure (B.P.), Respiratory Rate (R.R.) and Intensity of Ataxia Action (shaded area) in an Unanesthetized Dog.

No significant influence upon the pulse rate is seen after a large dose of cannabidiol. It lowers the blood pressure and the respiration markedly, but only for a short period (less than twenty minutes). Tetrahydrocannabinol, in a moderate dose, lowered the pulse rate by about 25 per cent for a short initial period, but in the course of the subsequent half-hour, in which the ataxia action reaches its peak, a very considerable increase in pulse rate, almost 100 per cent, took place. The maximum increase is only to a small extent due to the additional red oil administered forty minutes after the tetrahydrocannabinol. A large dose of tetrahydrocannabinol, injected at the peak of this effect, was followed by a decrease in pulse rate, from which it recovered to its former maximum rate about ninety minutes later at the time when the ataxia action was fully developed. The result of a subsequent dose of a synthetic homolog of hexahydrocannabinol, representing about 1 unit/Kg. of ataxia potency, is not entirely conclusive, but it suggests that the initial decrease in pulse rate does not occur if a small dose is administered when the pulse rate is high.

The increase in pulse rate is accompanied by reciprocal change in the respiratory rate and in blood pressure, but lags behind either of these changes. In a narcotized dog (60 mg. sodium amytal, intravenously; see Figure 6) only the initial decrease in pulse rate was observed. In non-narcotized cats, no increase in pulse rate was observed after any dose of tetrahydrocannabinol.

According to these findings, an increase in pulse rate in the dog is characteristic of moderate ataxia-effective doses of tetrahydro-

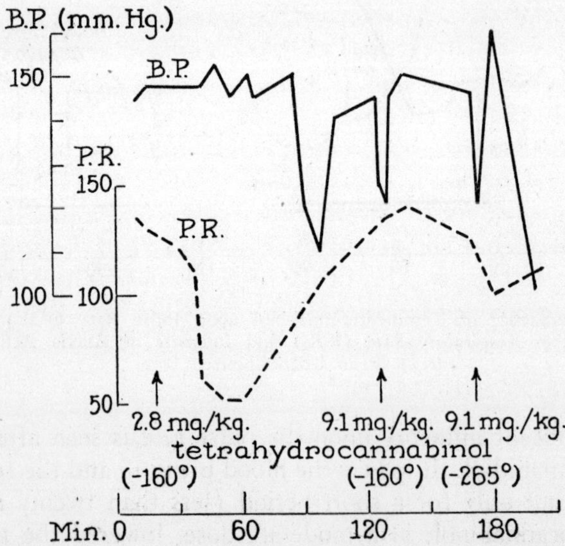

FIGURE 6.—Influence of Tetrahydrocannabinol upon Pulse Rate (P.R.) and Blood Pressure (B.P.) in an Anesthetized Dog.

cannabinol, and is closely correlated in time with the ataxia action. The present experiments suggest that the increased pulse rate is secondary to a depressing influence of the drug upon the blood pressure and respiration. This syndrome and its abolition by narcosis are indicative of a central origin and do not suggest a peripheral atropine-like mechanism. The emetic action also emphasizes the difference between marihuana and atropine; further, the pupil became increasingly small with the increase in pulse rate after the medium dose and showed a marked miosis at the peak of the ataxia action following the second dose of tetrahydrocannabinol (see Figure 5).

Central Stimulant Actions

A variety of symptoms of excitation can be observed after marihuana as well as from pure tetrahydrocannabinols. A picture resembling convulsant spasms may develop, especially in "tense" animals. More pronounced convulsive attacks are observed, in certain instances, as after combinations of marihuana with subthreshold doses of a hypnotic (amytal) or a central stimulant (benzedrine). Whereas all these phenomena are irregular effects of tetrahydrocannabinol in the dog, 7-methyl-tetrahydrocannabinol (LII; Table 50, No. 35) is outstanding among all the representatives of the cannabinol class because it always elicits a concomitance of ataxia and convulsions. Both manifestations are about parallel in intensity after intravenous administration to dogs. The stimulant action begins with hyperexcitability; touch releases short attacks of clonic tremor. At doses of greater ataxia effect, chronic convulsions are initiated by abrupt movements apparently tending to catch the dropping head or to counteract the swaying of the body. In the cat, the ataxia effect was not accompanied by convulsions.

Tetrahydrocannabidiol (LI), a derivative in the cannabidiol class, deserves a brief report because of its genuinely convulsant action. It is one of the reduction products of cannabidiol prepared by Adams, the presence of which in marihuana is not probable. Like cannabidiol and dihydrocannabidiol, it is devoid of ataxia action. Intravenous doses of about 50 mg./Kg. cause vigorous clonic-tonic, and, in some instances, strychnine-like convulsions followed by death. In intravenous doses from 10 to 18 mg./Kg., the manifestations are limited to fibrillary tremor and moderate excitation. Higher doses produce enormous degrees of respiratory and psychic excitation and clonic convulsions very similar to those produced by 7-methyltetrahydrocannabinol but of a faster rhythm. In a narrow range of dosage (about 18 to 21 mg./Kg.) and in certain strains of dogs, the convulsant action may be restricted to the muscles of the neck. A very specific effect is then produced consisting of periodic attacks of rhythmic, nodding movements of the head alone at a rate of two or three per second.* All symptoms begin only after a period of latency of thirty to seventy minutes after intravenous injection; this suggests a possible slow conversion into the convulsant agent. In cats and rabbits the $L.D._{50}$ is similar to that of the dog (cat: $>28<46$ mg./Kg.; rabbit: ± 40 mg./Kg.), death is rapid (three to five minutes after injection) even after threshold doses.

Structure-Activity Relation in the Cannabinol Class

A summary of the data on the ataxia activity of the pure cannabinols is given in Table 50. It can be seen that the entire group of hydrocannabinols is effective. The maximum effectiveness was found in the sub-group of tetrahydrocannabinols (Table 50, No. 3-19). The hexahydrocannabinols, however, were also effective, and not less than some of the tetrahydrocannabinols (No. 20-23). The dihydrocannabinols also appear to be effective, although we have not had the opportunity of testing them. One of them, prepared by Bergel et al.,[22] showed a potency estimated to be approximately 0.5.

Related groups of chemicals, namely, the aromatic non-hydrogenated cannabinols as well as the isomeric diphenyls containing no pyran bridge, the cannabidiols, are devoid of ataxia activity. However, other related substances, such as the 2,2-dimethyl-5-hydroxy-7-*n*-amyl-benzopyrans with open alkyl chains in positions 3 or 3 and 4, which represent simplified cannabinols in which carbon ring A is missing, still possess ataxia activity. The potency of these compounds (Nos. 26 and 27) is very low (0.03-0.04), and the effect is less specific inasmuch as these compounds do not have the large margin of safety characteristic of the active compounds from the cannabinol group. Doses only a little higher than the threshold dose of ataxia effect are in the lethal range. Connecting the 3,4-side-chains at the pyran ring so as to form a third ring increases the

*Shown in the motion picture of marihuana action edited by the U. S. Bureau of Narcotics and this department, 1939.

margin of safety and the potency. This is exemplified not only by the 3,4-tetramethylene- and methyl-3,4-tetramethylene derivatives of the same benzopyran (No. 32 and Nos. 33, 34 and 16), but also by the pentamethylene derivative, that is, the cycloheptane analog of apo-tetrahydrocannabinol (LIII; No. 25; potency 0.2).

In the group of tetrahydrogenated cannabinols there are enormous differences in potency. A study of these differences is of interest in relation to the details of structure of the tetrahydrocannabinol molecule essential for maximum ataxia activity.

The properties to be considered are:

1) The position of the double bonds in ring A.
2) Number and position of the methyl groups.
3) The alkyl groups at the pyran ring.
4) The amyl group.*

The position of the double bonds is of the greatest importance for the degree of activity. It must be concluded from the potencies of synthetic tetrahydrocannabinols that a conjugate position of the double bond, even in a laevo-rotatory isomer, results in products having not more than one-fourth the potency of those with non-conjugated bonds. However, in spite of great differences in optical rotation, whether non-conjugated double bonds are in the 7,8 or in the 8,9 position is not important. The position of the double bonds in natural products of maximum potency has yet to be ascertained.

The meta position of the methyl group in ring A appears to be important. In isomers having the methyl group in position ortho (No. 33) or para (No. 34) the potency is considerably lower than in the synthetic meta-methyl isomer (No. 16) and not markedly higher than in homologs of the latter (No. 32 and 39) in which the methyl group is missing or replaced by an ethyl group. On the other hand,

*A fifth factor of significance in the specific activity is the 1-hydroxyl group. Blocking of this group has a variable effect. Acetylated natural tetrahydrocannabinols are not markedly less potent than the free alcohols, whereas the acetates of synthetic isomers (see Table 50, Nos. 28 and 29) exhibited only 10 per cent or even less of the potency of the alcohols. Hydrolysis of even the highly potent esters resulted invariably in a product of lower potency. The rates of hydrolysis in the body and of the elimination of the alcoholic cleavage product are factors which complicate the interpretation of differences in potency between the alcohols and the acetates. The results from the more stable ethers (Table 7, Nos. 30 and 31) are of greater significance in showing that an open hydroxyl group is important. Recently a 2-hydroxyl isomer of 7,8,9,10-tetrahydrocannabinol was found to be "ineffective" in producing areflexia (Russell et al.),[81] and Alles and collaborators[74] found "no significant marihuana activity" from oral administration of synthetic hydroxyl-free tetrahydrocannabinols with and without the 9-methyl group.

introduction of a second *m*-methyl group into position 7 of synthetic tetrahydrocannabinol has no considerable influence upon the potency (No. 35), whereas it is decreased by introduction of a second methyl group at other positions (Nos. 36 and 37) even more than by a 9-ethyl in the place of methyl (No. 38). As in the case of the 9-alkyl group, lengthening of the 6,6-alkyl groups weakens the potency considerably (Nos. 39 and 40) but does not destroy it entirely. We have had no opportunity to examine tetrahydrocannabinols in which one or both of the 6,6-methyl groups are absent.

A particularly complete investigation has been possible on the significance of the amyl group at ring B. As is seen in the section on the chemistry of the tetrahydrocannabinols, there were available

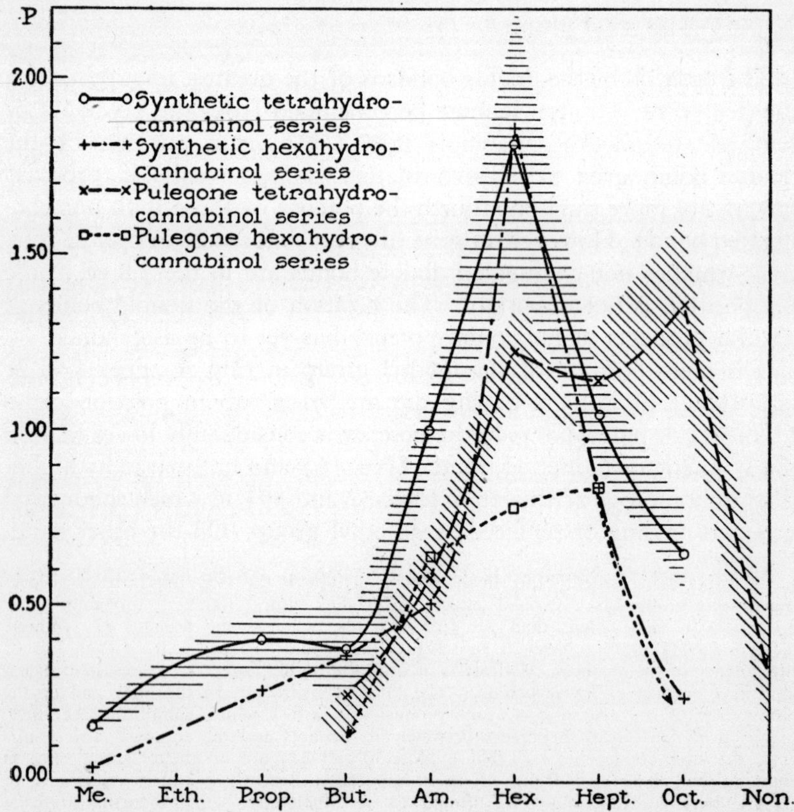

FIGURE 7.—Variation in Ataxia Potency (ordinate) in four Series of 3-Alkyl Homologs of Hydrocannabinols.

compounds in which the amyl group is substituted by straight alkyl chains of almost any number of carbon atoms between 0 and 9. Further, we have a homologous series of synthetic tetrahydrocannabinol, of the pulegone isomer, and of their reduction products, that is, two types of hexahydrocannabinols. An illustrative presentation of the results is given in Figure 7 through a graphic representation of the variation of potency with the length of the alkyl group.

In one of these four series of homologs the assay begins with the basic substance with no alkyl substitution in the 3-position (No. 47). It shows that absence of the alkyl chain decreases the potency enormously. Low potencies were found throughout in all four series in the homologs with shorter side chains, up to and including the butyl group. From then on the potency rises, but it is evident from the graph that in all four series the hexyl derivative is definitely more potent than the homologous isomer of the natural product with the amyl side chain. In three out of the four series, this increase in potency from the amyl to the hexyl derivative amounts to about 100 per cent or more (82, 265, and 110 per cent, respectively). With further lengthening of the side chain, a marked divergence occurs between the pulegone series and the three other series of hydrocannabinols. In all three latter series the potency drops and reaches a low level at the octyl derivatives. The heptyl derivatives are also considerably less potent than the hexyl derivatives except in the two pulegone series: hexyl and heptyl derivatives are equal in potency in the pulegone tetrahydrocannabinol series, and in the case of the reduced pulegone series there is no significant difference between the amyl, hexyl and heptyl derivatives. In the pulegone series, however, the drop in potency is only between the octyl and nonyl derivatives, with the octyl derivative possessing the maximum potency.*

Since none of the natural tetrahydrocannabinols appears to con-

---

*A related problem, namely, that of the significance of attaching to the phenol ring similar 3-side-chains by a different linkage, is raised by recent investigations (1942). Two groups of investigators synthesized analogous dibenzopyrans containing a 3-hydroxyl group, and attached aliphatic chains by ether- or esterification, that is, over a ≡C-O-C- instead of the natural ≡C-C- linkage. Alles et al.[75] found the 3-butyl and 3-butyryl derivatives devoid of ataxia effect, but unfortunately these analogs were lacking the 1-hydroxyl and in some cases also the 9-methyl group. Moreover, Alles's test method (oral administration) makes it difficult to evaluate substances of low potency. The studies of Bergel et al.[76] refer to the 3-*n*-butyl-, -amyl-, -hexyl- and -heptyloxy analogs of tetrahydrocannabinol. The hexyloxy homolog was the only one to show "feeble activity in 10-20 mg./Kg. doses," but unfortunately only the rabbit areflexia test was applied.

tain a side chain other than amyl, one is tempted to conclude from observations on those four homologous series that nature has not selected the most potent representative of the class and that the laboratory can synthesize structures of higher potency than nature. This conclusion would be premature because, so far, our findings refer only to synthetic isomers which, in some respects, differ markedly from the natural isomers. It will have to be determined whether the tetrahydrocannabinols with non-conjugated double bonds and high specific rotation are also more potent when they carry a longer side chain in position 3.

It is tempting to consider the significance of the spatial arrangement of the tetrahydrocannabinols in relation to their potency, particularly since the structure of those natural tetrahydrocannabinols which are superior in potency to the semi-synthetic isomers is as yet unknown. There is a marked difference between the synthetic tetrahydrocannabinols with the conjugated double bond, that is, with a pyran ring, and the natural and semi-synthetic tetrahydrocannabinols with a non-conjugated double bond, which, as well as the hexahydrocannabinols, are derivatives of dihydropyran. In the case of the pyrans the entire skeleton is arranged in one plane, whereas in the case of the dihydropyrans the planes of ring A and of ring B are divergent. But a still greater variety of spatial arrangements is disclosed by a stricter consideration of the four types specified on page 168. In type 1 (conjugated double bond), all three rings are in one plane, and isomerism is due only to asymmetry of C-atom 9. Both in type 2 (8,9 and 9,10) and type 4 (7,8), there is one out of two sub-groups in which the plane of ring A is tilted toward that of ring B, either with (type 4) or without (type 2) simultaneous asymmetry in position 9. In other isomers, however, ring A extends through two (type 3) or even three planes (the other sub-groups of types 2 and 4), in types 3 and 4 with simultaneous asymmetry in position 9, but not in type 2. It may be noted that out of the three laevogyrous isomers synthesized by Adams the one with a tilted A-plane (8,9; –265°; P=7.3)—in which the laevorotation in position 9 of the starting material, *l*-cannabidiol, was abolished by the shift of the double bond into 8,9—is not less potent than one which, in addition, has an asymmetry in position 9 (7,8; –130°; P=6.5). On the other hand, both possess more than three times the potency of the isomer having asymmetry only in position 9 (conjugated; –114°; P = 1.66). Nevertheless, optical activity at this position is not irrelevant, as is indicated by the difference between the potencies of the *d*- and the *l*-isomer in the latter instance (0.38 versus 1.66). At any rate, the existence of such a variety of arrangements in space may help to explain the difficulties in obtaining products of reproducible specific rotation and potency, and perhaps also the failures in effecting crystallization. The interest of the pharmacologist will be focused on the question of the spatial arrangement correlated with the exceptional potencies of the natural isomers which apparently originate from the same *l*-cannabidiol which *in vitro* condenses to a product only about half as potent.

Participation of the Different Active Principles of Different Actions of Crude Marihuana Preparations

There are many indications that the pharmacological actions of the individual active principles are not identical with those of the crude drug and that the individual components have a variable share in the composite activity of the crude material. This is best demonstrated by the potency indices of the pure substances. Table 51 reviews the potencies of various impure and pure products on the basis of the three main effects of marihuana,—ataxia, corneal areflexia and synergistic sleep-prolongation,—and, in its last two columns, the potency indices comparing ataxia and areflexia, and ataxia and synergistic hypnotic effectiveness. If the activity of all these

Table 51

Potency indices

Preparation	I	II	III	IV	V
	Relative potency, determined by			Ratio I/II	Ratio I/III
	Ataxia test (dog)	Corneal areflexia test (rabbit)	Synerg. hypnotic test (mouse)		
American red oil	1.00	1.00	1.00	1.00	1.00
Oriental red oil	2.00	0.46	—	4.30	—
U.S.P. fluidextract	0.014	0.0065	—	2.10	—
Semi-synthetic tetrahydrocannabinol (−165°)	2.10	0.30	<0.63	7.00	>3.33
Semi-synthetic tetrahydrocannabinol (−160°)	1.90	0.14	—	13.00	—
Crystall. cannabidiol	<0.013	<0.005	3.10	—	<0.004
Cannabinol	0	0	0	—	—

products were due to one and the same principle, the potency indices should be constant throughout. Instead, they vary and are particularly divergent when highly purified, chemically homogeneous substances are employed. Thus, the potency index virtually is $\frac{1}{\infty}$ in the comparison of ataxia and synergistic hypnotic action of cannabidiol, which is a clear expression of the fact that cannabidiol is responsible for the latter action and takes no share in other aspects of marihuana action. Similarly, the relationship between ataxia and areflexia action is expressed by the high potency index of highly purified semi-synthetic tetrahydrocannabinol, pointing to an almost exclusive ataxia effect. The lower value in the case of the less completely purified substance could indicate that a by-product with areflexia activity accompanies the ataxia-effective tetrahydrocannabinol. This may be the same substance which is accumulated in the distillate oil (potency index: 1.0), when it is prepared from a crude extract having a potency index of 2.1. The divergencies of the three potency indices of ataxia and synergistic hypnotic action may be explained by the presence of cannabidiol in the distillate oil as well as in the incompletely purified tetrahydrocannabinol that was obtained by condensation of cannabidiol.

It is clear that the potency indices give numerical proof that the three main actions of marihuana are represented by different principles, tetrahydrocannabinol, cannabidiol and an unknown principle, whereas cannabinol exerts none of these actions. The only reservation necessary with regard to this statement is that, due to the lack of a reliable quantitative method for measuring the areflexia potency, the areflexia and ataxia principles have not been differentiated with absolute certainty.

A more explicit answer to the question of the correlation between ataxia and areflexia action is made possible by recent work:*

Publications of the Manchester investigators[76, 79, 81] show how they use the corneal areflexia test for quantitative purposes, and also supply data on the "areflexia potency," among others, of thirteen substances the ataxia potencies of which had been determined in our department. Thus, the areflexia/ataxia potency indices of a considerable group of substances become available. Designating them by the number under which they are recorded in our Table 50 and giving in parenthesis the Manchester areflexia and the Cornell ataxia

*The following paragraphs of this section were added after the completion of the manuscript. November 1943.

potencies the results are as follows: No. 16 (standard; 1/1); No. 10 (5/9.3); No. 17 (0.15/0.38); No. 21 (0.3/0.5); No. 26 ($<$0.07/0.33); No. 32 ($>$0.2/0.126); No. 42 ($<$0.05/0.16); No. 43 ($<$0.05/0.4); No. 44 (1/0.38); No. 45 (10/1.82); No. 46 (10/1.05); No. 47 (1/0.66); and No. 33 from Table 6 (1/8.66). Whereas in two instances the potency indices may be found close to 1.0, all others vary widely,—between $<$0.12 and 9.3, the highest value being 80 times the lowest. The mean of the group is 1.92 with a variance of 7.43 and a coefficient of variation $\pm$142.

A majority of the areflexia potency determinations reported by the Manchester group appear to be based upon only one or two experiments and they therefore do not have the reliability of the assays on dogs, and must be regarded as not more than a rough approximation. The ratios therefore must be accepted with reservation, but taken at their face value their great variability indicates that corneal areflexia results from the action of an unknown substance differing from the tetrahydrocannabinols causing ataxia in dogs.

This conclusion is supported by the work of Alles and collaborators (1942),[74] who showed that gentle oxidation destroys the areflexia activity, whereas the ataxia principles are stable. Similarly Russell and collaborators showed[58] that ultraviolet irradiation destroys the areflexia principle, whereas according to our experiments (see page 187) the ataxia principles are not influenced by this treatment.

VI. Some Other Pharmacological Aspects of Marihuana

While these studies have been primarily concerned with the characteristics of the active principles of marihuana, some information has been obtained on a number of other aspects of the pharmacology of marihuana, a brief discussion of which will conclude this report.

Stability

Due to their failure to isolate the active principles of marihuana and to the great differences in the potency of different preparations, earlier investigators concluded that they were unstable. Upon this assumption the sale of a hashish in some parts of India[32] is limited by governmental regulation to preparations less than one year old. No such limitation has been found necessary for therapeutic preparations of cannabis. This difference may be due to the conditions determining chemical alterations, for an understanding of which a knowledge of the chemical nature of the active principles is essential.

We found that the hemp herb which had been stacked in the open for several years had undiminished potency; a type of exposure obviously not favorable for chemical alteration of tetrahydrocannabinols. Nor could we find deterioration of distillate oils preserved for considerable periods of time. For example, a comparative bioassay was made with two batches of our standard redistillate oil, one of which had been preserved under seal at low temperature, and the other exposed to the air in an open container at room temperature for two years. The potency of the two batches was the same within the limits of accuracy of the ataxia method.

Circumstances affecting the stability became manifest when tetrahydrocannabinols were bioassayed before and after acetylation. Natural tetrahydrocannabinol acetate lost about 50 per cent of its potency when hydrolyzed in a strongly alkaline medium. Oxidation is thus found to be a major factor responsible for deterioration and is greatly favored in solution and at an alkaline reaction, as is the case with other aromatic alcohols. Pure tetrahydrocannabinols, synthetic as well as natural, when in a neutral alcoholic solution, preserved in a refrigerator and air excluded, were stable over a period of years.

Duration of Action and Mode of Administration

The time relations of marihuana action in dogs have two interesting features: the duration is long even after threshold doses, with intravenous as well as oral administration, and so are the periods of latency and of the development of action.

The action lasts considerably longer after oral than after intravenous administration. The ataxia effect of a threshold dose has already declined an hour after intravenous administration, but not before the end of the second hour after oral administration. This was established from the earlier experiments with crude preparations, but has now been confirmed with pure substances from the cannabinol class. Thus the period of latency of the ataxia action—at least five to ten minutes after intravenous and at least twenty minutes after oral administration—is not decreased when pure tetrahydrocannabinols are used.

The ratio between intravenous and oral effectiveness of pure tetrahydrocannabinols, when determined intra-individually in carefully calibrated dogs, was >10, >10, >10, >10, >25, <44, that is, about 30. Walton found about 10.0 for distillate oils.[65, 66] This indicates that the difference between oral and intravenous doses may be greater in pure substances.

The problems of the relative effectiveness and the duration of the period of latency are of particular interest in connection with marihuana smoking. Many authors reported that the smoker notices the effects of marihuana almost at once. These statements are confirmed by the statements of many addicts which we reviewed in about five hundred questionnaires collected by the U. S. Bureau of Narcotics. The period of latency must therefore be ascribed to a process of mobilization of the active substance rather than to the conversion of the substance administered into an effective form. Low solubility and a slow rate of solution in water delay the onset of the effect after intravenous as well as oral administration, whereas these factors are less influential after inhalation.

A few experiments were conducted to find out whether the intensity or the time relations of the effects of pure active substances were influenced by the presence of inert substances from the raw material. The effect of the combination of cannabidiol with tetrahydrocannabinol was compared with that of tetrahydrocannabinol alone. No difference was observed in the potency nor in any other feature of the ataxia action.

Tolerance, Habituation, Addiction

Changes in the individual sensitivity to a drug, which have a bearing on the problems of tolerance, habituation, or addiction, can only be studied under experimental circumstances faithfully emulating those of the habitual use of the drug in man, namely uninterrupted daily administration. Animals used for purposes of bioassay of the drug of necessity receive their doses by an entirely different schedule, because the intervals must be long enough to exclude after-effects from the preceding dose upon the effect of the new dose. Although our dogs have been used for bioassays over long periods of time, up to almost three years, they have no value for studies on habituation.

The data obtained on intra-individual variations in sensitivity (Table 49) must be used with this reservation. They indicate beyond doubt that even prolonged treatment, by the procedure employed in repeated bioassay experiments, does not necessarily produce a decrease in sensitivity and never produces a change characteristic of genuine habituation. On the contrary, there is actually an increase in sensitivity in many animals. Moreover, the apparent decrease in sensitivity observed in some animals can be explained (see page 179) by the phenomenon of over-compensation of the ataxia symptoms. This is of the type of an "efferent" adaptation to the drug effect, whereas genuine habituation is due either to afferent adaptation to the drug action, namely adaptation of absorption or metabolism, or to cellular adaptation at the site of the cellular attack of the drug.

Synergism of Marihuana and the Problem of the Mechanism of Marihuana Action

Most important among the numerous unsolved problems of the pharmacology of marihuana is the question of the mechanism of its central nervous actions. Superficial similarity to the opiates and even less justified comparisons with the hypnotics have been the basis for interpreting these central actions as manifestations of a depressant influence upon the higher nervous centers. The only attempt to analyze the marihuana mechanism experimentally (Joel[44]) was apparently based on the assumption of a stimulatory mechanism. Joel tried to localize the site of the ataxia action by comparing the effects in normal, decorticated, and decerebrated cats. Normal cats show swaying, decrease in motility, cataleptic perseverance and general inhibition. Swaying was the only symptom in thalamic cats. No effect at all was seen in decerebrated cats. "In view of the relative intactness of the postural regulations located in midbrain and medulla" Joel interprets his findings as suggestive evidence that marihuana "acts preponderantly upon the hemispheres." Indeed, his observations show that the action of marihuana does not interfere with postural regulations and that, if the ataxia is due to a stimulatory influence, the site of the stimulation is higher than the red nucleus and even the thalamus. If, however, the marihuana effects are due to a depressant action, Joel's experiments are less conclusive.

A different approach to the problem of the mechanism may be seen in some of our experiments. They were planned to find out how drugs from other pharmacological groups—hypnotics (amytal) and stimulants (benzedrine)—influence the marihuana action.

The results of experiments with combinations of amytal and marihuana are summarized in Table 52. The hypnotic alone was capable of producing ataxia; only on closer inspection can the rhythm of swaying be distinguished from that due to marihuana. The amytal ataxia was produced by doses well below the threshold of hypnotic effectiveness. Marihuana exerted no synergistic hypnotic influence. Nor was a hypnotic influence of amytal manifested by a decrease of the ataxia symptoms. Rather the ataxia in some of the experiments was increased, as expressed by a somewhat longer duration of the effects.

TABLE 52

Synergism of amytal and marihuana in the dog

Animal No.	Dose of		Effect			Duration of ataxia action min.	Ataxia potency of combination ref. to same dose of marihuana alone
	Marihuana standard Mg./Kg.	Amytal sodium Mg./Kg.	Excitation	Hypnosis	Ataxia grade		
78	—	9.7	—	—	III–IV	>5 <42	2.5 ± 0.4
78	0.96	9.7	++	—	III–IV	>124	2.5 ± 0.4
72	—	16.3	—	—	IV	>60 <110	±3.0
72	0.82	16.3	convulsions	—	IV	>105	±3.0
85	—	18.7	—	—	IV–V	>38 <89	>1.5
85	5.00	18.7	convulsions	—	IV–V	>75	>1.5
64	0.54	6.1	—	—	II	brief	<2.0
73	3.81	6.3	—	—	III–IV	<93	3.3
84	6.70	6.7	—	—	III–IV	>51 <103	5.0
52	1.44	7.2	—	—	III–IV	>75 <125	3.0
71	0.60	7.6	—	—	II	>44 <104	>2.5
22	1.05	8.0	—	—	III–IV	>35 <60	2.2 ± 0.7

Benzedrine-marihuana experiments are presented in Table 53. Benzedrine, when given alone, was devoid of any noticeable effect. In combination with marihuana, a remarkable synergism was manifest; in the presence of benzedrine, marihuana was 1.8 to 2.4 times as effective as in preceding calibration experiments in the same animals.

Thus, four observations are available which contribute to the explanation of the mechanism of action of marihuana: (a) Marihuana ataxia is abolished by the elimination of the higher levels of the brain (Joel). (b) An ataxia similar in all features to that produced by marihuana results from the destruction of the cerebellum

TABLE 53

Synergism of benzedrine and marihuana in the dog

Animal No.	Dose of		Effect			Ataxia potency of combination ref. to same dose of marihuana alone
	Marihuana standard Mg./Kg.	Benzedrine Mg./Kg.	Time interval to vomiting min.	Excitation	Ataxia grade	
25	4.04	—	∞	—	II	—
25	8.04	—	11	—	IV	—
25	8.64	—	∞	—	III	—
25	9.45	—	∞	—	III	—
25	—	0.207	7	—	0	0
25	3.46	0.229	13	+	III	}2.35±0.35
25	4.04	0.229	10	convulsions	IV	
72	1.70	—	∞	—	II–(III)	—
72	2.31	—	∞	—	II–III	—
72	2.71	—	∞	—	III	—
72	—	0.200	8	—	0	0
72	0.87	0.200	5	convulsions	II–III	2.40±0.40
84	5.00	—	∞	—	III	—
84	8.00	—	∞	—	(III)–IV	—
84	—	0.150	∞	—	0	0
84	3.50	0.150	∞	+	(III)–IV	1.85±0.45

(human pathology and extirpation experiments in the dog). (c) Marihuana ataxia is not markedly influenced by low doses of a hypnotic. (d) Marihuana ataxia is markedly increased by subthreshold doses of a stimulant of higher cerebral centers.

These observations are not sufficient to form any conception of the mechanism of action. If it were permissible to use them for developing a tentative working hypothesis, such an attempt might be based upon the rather meager evidence suggesting that marihuana ataxia has two prerequisites: (1) Primary impulses of suprathalamic or supranuclear origin which tend to cause *incoordinated* motor effects. (2) Regulating impulses of cerebellar origin which tend to restore *coordinated* muscular activity. Marihuana action, on this hypothesis, would then result in a preponderance of incoordinated suprathalamic activity over the regulating cerebellar control, either by depressing the latter or by stimulating the former. Further experiments are required to decide whether the rôle of marihuana is that of a stimulant or of a depressant and whether the site of action is supranuclear or cerebellar. Studies of the influence of decerebration and of marihuana in decerebellated dogs should help in further analysis.

SUMMARY

1. This review of the pharmacology of marihuana is centered around the chemical and pharmacological identification of the active principles of hemp. Coordination of chemical and pharmacological investigations as a prerequisite to success in the search for unknown principles and of the analysis of the structure-activity relationship of these compounds is discussed.

2. In a survey of the sources of preparations with marihuana activity, hemp seeds are disclosed as a heretofore unknown source of active substances.

3. Varieties of hemp can be distinguished according to genotypic differences of the content of active principles which persist over generations independently of soil and climate.

4. The pharmacological actions of marihuana are analyzed with regard to their specificity and their usefulness as indicators of specific components.

5. Sixty-five substances from the new class of cannabinols and related classes are reviewed, among which are the essential components of the marihuana-active hemp oils. The discovery of this class, the synthesis of these representatives, and their structural elucidation led the way to the discovery of the active substances.

6. Quantitative assay procedures are described for the most important marihuana effects that are observed in the animal experiment. The assay of the ataxia effect in the dog and of the synergistic hypnotic effect in the mouse with refined procedures are shown to be reliable expedients for measuring these two marihuana actions, whereas the areflexia effect in rabbits failed to show the reproducibility required for quantitative purposes.

7. With the aid of these methods the natural tetrahydrocannabinols are shown to be active principles responsible for ataxia in dogs and psychic action in man. They are intermediate products between the two ineffective substances which compose the bulk of hemp oil: a labile excretion product of the plant, cannabidiol, and a stable end-product, cannabinol. The conversion of cannabidiol into active tetrahydrocannabinol by a natural environmental influence has been paralleled by ultraviolet irradiation *in vitro.*

8. Numerous isomers, homologs and analogs of tetra- and hexahydrocannabinol are shown to possess the specific marihuana action.

The potency varies enormously and is highest in natural, optically active—laevogyrous—tetrahydrocannabinols.

9. The significance of many of the structural details of the tetrahydrocannabinol molecule for marihuana activity is elucidated by quantitative determinations of relative potency. Special attention was devoted to a study of the importance of variations in the length of the 3-alkyl side chain of tetrahydrocannabinols. In studying methyl to nonyl homologs of the original amyl derivative occurring in nature, it was found that the maximum potency is not at the amyl, but at the hexyl homolog, and in two out of four homologous series at the representatives with still longer side chains.

10. In addition to the ataxia and the psychic action, other pharmacological attributes of the tetrahydrocannabinols are a decrease in the respiratory and an increase in the pulse rates in the non-narcotized dog.

11. The synergistic hypnotic action of marihuana in the mouse is to be attributed to the otherwise inert cannabidiol.

12. The corneal areflexia action in the rabbit was much stronger in impure distillate oils than in pure tetrahydrocannabinols, which leads to the conclusion that this action is either poorly reproducible or must be attributed to a different, as yet unknown, principle.

13. Only one among the numerous cannabinol derivatives, 7-methyltetrahydrocannabinol, was found to produce a motor stimulant—convulsant—action concomitant with ataxia action. A cannabidiol derivative, tetrahydrocannabidiol, was found to have very specific convulsant action in the dog.

14. A central stimulant (benzedrine) considerably increased the ataxia action of marihuana, whereas a hypnotic (amytal) had no influence.

BIBLIOGRAPHY

1. Adams: Science, *92,* 115, 1940.
2. Adams, Hunt and Clark: Jour. Amer. Chem. Soc., *62,* 196, 1940.
3. Adams, Cain and Wolff: Jour. Amer. Chem. Soc., *62,* 732, 1940.
4. Adams, Hunt and Clark: Jour. Amer. Chem. Soc., *62,* 735, 1940.
5. Adams, Wolff, Cain and Clark: Jour. Amer. Chem. Soc., *62,* 1770, 1940.
6. Adams, Pease and Clark: Jour. Amer. Chem. Soc., *62,* 2194, 1940.
7. Adams, Pease, Clark and Baker: Jour. Amer. Chem. Soc., *62,* 2197, 1940.
8. Adams, Cain and Baker: Jour. Amer. Chem. Soc., *62,* 2201, 1940.
9. Adams, Baker and Wearn: Jour. Amer. Chem. Soc., *62,* 2204, 1940.
10. Adams and Baker: Jour. Amer. Chem. Soc., *62,* 2208, 1940.

11. Adams, Wolff, Cain and Clark: Jour. Amer. Chem. Soc., *62,* 2215, 1940.
12. Adams, Pease, Cain, Baker, Clark, Wolff, Wearn and Loewe: Jour. Amer. Chem. Soc., *62,* 2245, 1940.
13. Adams, Pease, Cain and Clark: Jour. Amer. Chem. Soc.,*62,* 2402, 1940.
14. Adams and Baker: Jour. Amer. Chem. Soc., *62,* 2405, 1940.
15. Adams, Loewe, Pease, Cain, Wearn, Baker and Wolff: Jour. Amer. Chem. Soc., *62,* 2566, 1940.
16. Adams, Loewe, Jellinek and Wolff: Jour. Amer. Chem. Soc., *63,* 1971, 1941.
17. Adams, Smith and Loewe: Jour. Amer. Chem. Soc., *63,* 1973, 1941.
18. Adams, Cain and Loewe: Jour. Ameri. Chem. Soc., *63,* 1977, 1941.
19. Adams, Cain, McPhee and Wearn: Jour. Amer. Chem. Soc., *63,* 2209, 1941.
20. Adams, Loewe, Smith and McPhee: Jour. Amer. Chem. Soc.,*64,* 694, 1942.
21. Balozet: League of Nations, O.C./Cannabis/1542, 1937.
22. Bergel and Wagner: Annalen d. Chem., *482,* 55, 1930.
23. Bergel, Todd and Work: Chem. Industry, 86, 1938.
24. Bembry and Powell: Jour. Amer. Chem. Soc., *63,* 2766, 1941.
25. Blatt: Jour. Wash. Acad. Sci., *28,* 465, 1938.
26. Bouquet: League of Nations, O.C./Cannabis/14, 1939.
27. Bouquet: League of Nations, O.C., 1545 (c), 1937.
28. Buergi: Deutsch. Med. Wochenschr., 1924, No. 45.
29. Cahn: Jour. Chem. Soc., 1342, 1932.
30. Cahn: Jour. Chem. Soc., 1400, 1933.
31. Casparis and Baur: Pharm. Acta Helv., *2,* 107, 1927.
32. Chopra and Chopra: Indian Jour. Med. Research Mem. (Mem. No. 31), p. 1, 1939.
33. Fraenkel: Arch. exp. Path. u. Pharmakol., *49,* 266, 1903.
34. Ghosh, Todd, Pascell and Wilkinson: Jour. Chem. Soc., 118, 1940.
35. Ghosh, Todd and Wilkinson: Jour. Chem. Soc., 118, 1940.
36. Ghosh, Todd and Wilkinson: Jour. Chem. Soc., 1393, 1940.
37. Ghosh, Todd and Wright: Jour. Chem. Soc., 137, 1941.
38. Gayer: Arch. exp. Path. u. Pharmakol., *129,* 312, 1928.
39. Goodall: Pharm. Jour. *84,* 112, 1910.
40. Haagen-Smit, Wawre, Koepfli, Alles, et al.: Science, *91,* 602, 1940.
41. Hare: Therap. Gazette, *11,* 225, 1887.
42. Houghton and Hamilton: Amer. Jour. Pharm., *80,* 16, 1908.
43. Jacob and Todd: Nature, *145,* 350, 1940; Jour. Chem. Soc., 649, 1940.
44. Joel: Pflügers Arch., *209,* 526, 1925.
45. Loewe: Jour. Pharmacol. and Exper. Therap., *66,* 23, 1939.
46. Loewe: Jour. Amer. Pharm. Assoc., *28,* 427, 1939.
47. Loewe: Jour. Amer. Pharm. Assoc., *29,* 162, 1940.
48. Loewe and Modell: Jour. Pharmacol. and Exper. Therap., *72,* 27, 1941.
49. Liautaud: Ac. Sc., 149, 1844.
50. Macdonald: Nature, *147,* 167, 1941.
51. Marx and Eckhardt: Arch. exp. Path. u. Pharmakol., *170,* 395, 1933.
52. Matchett, Levine, Benjamin, Robinson and Pope: Jour. Amer. Pharm. Assoc. *29,* 399, 1940.
53. Matchett and Loewe: Jour. Amer. Pharm. Assoc., *30,* 130, 1941.
54. Merz and Bergner: Arch. der Pharmaz., *278,* 49, 1940.
55. Powell, Salmon, Bembry and Walton: Science, *93,* 522, 1941.

56. Robinson: Jour. Amer. Pharm. Assoc., *30,* 616, 1941.
57. Robinson and Matchett: Jour. Amer. Pharm. Assoc., *29,* 448, 1940.
58. Russell, Todd, Wilkinson, Macdonald and Woolfe: (a) Jour. Chem. Soc., 169, 1941; (b) ibid. 826, 1941.
59. See: Deutsch, Med. Wochenschr., 679, 1890.
60. Todd: Nature, 829, 1940.
61. U. S. Treasury Dept.: Review of Progress on Marihuana Investigation during 1938.
62. U. S. Treasury Dept.: Marihuana: Its Identification, Washington, 1938.
63. U. S. Treasury Dept., Bureau of Narcotics: Report of the Marihuana Investigation, Summer 1937.
64. Viehoever: Amer. Jour. Pharmacy, *109,* No. 12, 1937.
65. Walton: Marihuana, Philadelphia-London, 1938.
66. Walton, Martin and Keller: Jour. Pharmacol. and Exper. Therap., *62,* 239, 1938.
67. Wiechowski: Arch. exp. Path. u. Pharmakol., *119,* 59, 1927.
68. Wollner, Matchett, Levine and Loewe: Jour. Amer. Chem. Soc., *64,* 26, 1942.
69. Wood, Barlow, Spivey and Easterfield: Jour. Chem. Soc., *69,* 539, 1896.
70. Wood, Barlow, Spivey and Easterfield: Jour. Chem. Soc., *75,* 20, 1899.
71. Work, Bergel and Todd: Biochem. Jour., *33,* 124, 1939.

ADDENDUM TO BIBLIOGRAPHY:*

72. Adams: Harvey Lectures, Ser. XXXVII, 1941-1942, p. 168.
73. Adams, Smith and Loewe: Jour. Amer. Chem. Soc., *64,* 2087, 1942.
74. Alles, Haagen-Smit, Feigen and Dendliker: Jour. Pharm. and Exp. Ther., 76, 21, 1942.
75. Alles, Icke and Feigen: Jour. Amer. Chem. Soc. *64,* 2031, 1942.
76. Bergel, Morrison, Rinderknecht, Todd, Macdonald and Woolfe: Jour. Chem. Soc., 286, 1943.
77. Fulton: Indust. & Engin. Chem., *14,* 407, 1942.
78. Hitzemann: Arch. der Pharmazie *276,* 353, 1941.
79. Leaf, Todd and Wilkinson: Jour. Chem. Soc., 185, 1942.
80. Madinaveitia, Russell and Todd: Jour. Chem. Soc., 628, 1942.
81. Russell, Todd, Wilkinson, Macdonald and Woolfe: Jour. Chem. Soc., 826, 1941.
82. Simonsen and Todd: Jour. Chem. Soc., 188, 1942.

*See footnote, page 150.

Summary

George B. Wallace, M.D., Chairman

The widespread publicity describing the dangerous effects of marihuana usage in New Orleans and other southern cities, especially among school children, had its repercussion in the city of New York, and some anxiety was experienced as to the possibility that similar conditions were present or might develop here. Because of this, Mayor La Guardia asked The New York Academy of Medicine for an opinion as to the advisability of studying the whole marihuana problem. The Academy recommended that such a study be made and outlined its scope in general terms. Following this, the Mayor appointed a committee empowered to make the study. This committee consisted of two internists, three psychiatrists, two pharmacologists, and one public health expert, and the Commissioners of Correction, of Health, and of Hospitals, and the Director of the Division of Psychiatry of the Department of Hospitals, ex officio.

The Committee formulated a plan for the study, and the expenses were arranged for through grants by the New York Foundation, the Friedsam Foundation and the Commonwealth Fund. The study was begun in April 1940.

The first phase of the study concerned the extent of marihuana smoking in New York City, its incidence among school children, its relation to crime, and its effects on individuals using it. For obtaining this information, the Commissioner of Police assigned to the Committee six police officers, four men and two women, who served as "plain clothes" investigators. These investigators circulated in the districts in which marihuana appeared to be most widely used, particularly Harlem, associated with marihuana users, and found out as much as possible about sources of supply, means of distribution, and effects of marihuana on users. Included in this survey were a careful watch on school children in both grade and high schools and interviews with school principals.

As a result of this investigation the Committee came to the conclusion that marihuana distribution and usage is found mainly in Harlem, the population of which is predominately Negro and Latin-American, and to a less extent in the Broadway area extending from 42nd to 59th Streets. The local supply comes from individual peddlers and from "tea-pads," which are establishments for marihuana smoking. There are no figures available as to the number of marihuana users in New York City, but a conservative estimate is that there are some 500 peddlers and 500 "tea-pads" in Harlem.

The marihuana users with whom contact was made in this study were persons without steady employment. The majority fall in the age group of 20 to 30 years. Idle and lacking initiative, they suffer boredom and seek distraction. Smoking is indulged in for the sake of conviviality and sociability and because it affords a temporary feeling of adequacy in meeting disturbing situations.

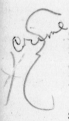

The confirmed user smokes from 6 to 10 cigarettes a day. The effects are easily recognized by the smoker, the desirable stage being what is known as "high." When this is reached, the smoking is stopped. If a "too high" state is reached, the taking of beverages such as beer or sweet soda pop, or a cold bath are considered effective countermeasures.

In most instances, the behavior of the smoker is of a friendly, sociable character. Aggressiveness and belligerency are not commonly seen, and those showing such traits are not allowed to remain in "tea-pads."

The marihuana user does not come from the hardened criminal class and there was found no direct relationship between the commission of crimes of violence and marihuana. "Tea-pads" have no direct association with houses of prostitution, and marihuana itself has no specific stimulant effect in regard to sexual desires.

There is no organized traffic in marihuana among New York City school children, and any smoking that occurs in this group is limited to isolated instances.

Smoking marihuana can be stopped abruptly with no resulting mental or physical distress comparable to that of morphine withdrawal in morphine addicts.

The second division of the study was the clinical one, the purpose of which was to ascertain the effects of marihuana on the individual user. There were two phases of this work, the general medical study and the psychological study. Wards in the municipal hospital on Welfare Island (now known as Goldwater Memorial Hospital) were made available by the Commissioner of Hospitals. The subjects for the study were drawn from the prison population at the Penitentiary on Riker's Island, as arranged by the Commissioner of Correction. They were under sentence for terms varying from three months to three years, most of them for what would be called minor criminal offenses. They volunteered for the study, the purpose and procedure of which had been fully explained to them. They were kept in the hospital in groups of 6 to 10, for a period of study of approximately a month. The subjects afforded the sample especially desired, for over half of them were marihuana smokers and the others of the class from which marihuana smokers come. The personnel conducting the study consisted of a physician in charge, with an assistant physician, three psychologists, and a secretary. The subjects were under the constant supervision of the medical staff, nurses and attendants.

In studying the effects of marihuana on the 77 subjects selected for the study, the drug was given either in the form of an extract taken by mouth, or was smoked in cigarettes. The dose given to produce definite systemic reactions ranged from a minimal one of 1 cc. to a maximum of 22 cc. of the extract, and from 1 to 10 cigarettes. The effects of smoking appeared immediately and usually passed off in from one to three or four hours. Those from the extract came on more gradually and persisted for a longer time, in some instances for twenty-four hours or more. As the dose for any individual was increased, the effects usually were more marked and of longer duration, but the effect of any given dose varied with the individual subjects.

Although some of the subjects became restless and talkative under marihuana influence, a mental state characterized by a sense of well-being, relaxation and unawareness of surroundings, followed by drowsiness, was present in most instances when the subject was left undisturbed. Generally, there was observed a difficulty in focusing and sustaining mental attention. In company, the subjects were lively and given to talkativeness, fits of laughter and good-natured joking. The pleasurable effects, classed as euphoric, were frequently interrupted or replaced by a state of apprehension of varying degree.

In a limited number of the subjects there were alterations in behavior giving rise to antisocial expression. This was shown by unconventional acts not permitted in public, anxiety reactions, opposition and antagonism, and eroticism. Effects such as these would be considered conducive to acts of violence. However, any tendency toward violence was expressed verbally and not by physical actions, and in no case was restraint by force needed.

In addition to its effect on mental states, physical symptoms resulting from the administration of marihuana were recorded. Of these, tremor, ataxia, dizziness, a sensation of floating in space, dilation of the pupils, dryness of the throat, nausea and vomiting, an urge to urinate, hunger, and a desire for sweets were the most striking. Tremor and ataxia and dizziness were of the greatest frequency. These symptoms may be disturbing to the subject, and if marked enough, cause anxiety and interrupt the euphoric state.

On some occasions, instead of the marihuana concentrate, preparations supplied by Dr. Roger Adams were given. These were tetrahydrocannabinol, made from cannabidiol, corresponding to a principle found in the plant, a synthetic tetrahydrocannabinol, an isomer of the natural one, and a synthetic hexyl-hydrocannabinol. They all produced effects similar in character to those from the concentrate. Their relative potency could be determined only approximately. The rough estimate was that 1 cc. of the concentrate had as its equivalent 15 mg. of the natural tetrahydrocannabinol, 60 mg. of the hexyl-hydrocannabinol, and 120 mg. of the synthetic tetrahydrocannabinol.

In the total group studied, what are known as psychotic episodes occurred in 9 of the subjects. In 6 instances, they were of short duration, persisting for from three to ten hours, and were characterized by mental confusion and excitement of a delirious nature with periods of laughter and of anxiety. These effects correspond to those often reported in marihuana literature and are examples of acute marihuana intoxication which in many ways is similar to acute alcoholic intoxication. In the other 3 cases, one subject had a mild psychotic reaction after smoking one cigarette. Later, a typical psychotic state came on four hours after the subject had taken tetrahydrocannabinol and persisted for six days. This subject subsequently was found to have a history of epileptic attacks so that the psychotic episode was probably related to epilepsy. The second subject had previously been a drug addict. She was given marihuana on several occasions, at times showing only euphoric effects and other times confusion and worriment. She left the hospital depressed and moody, and a week later was committed to a State hospital with the diagnosis of psychosis. After six months, she was discharged as cured. The third subject showed no unusual effects of marihuana which was given on several occasions during his stay at the hospital. Some days after his return to the penitentiary he developed a psychotic state diagnosed "Psychosis with psychopathic personality." This was considered an example of what is known as "prison psychosis," a condition which has been noted in persons emotionally unstable subjected to the depressing atmosphere of prison incarceration. The precise role of marihuana in the psychotic states in the three unstable subjects is not clear. In the case of the second and third subject, the fact that they were sent back to prison to complete their sentences must be considered an important if not the main factor in bringing on the psychosis.

In the clinical study of the effect of marihuana on functions of various organs of the body, there were found an increase in pulse rate and blood pressure and an increase in blood sugar and metabolic rate. No changes were found in the circulation rate and vital capacity. Tests on renal and liver function were negative. No changes were found in blood counts and hemoglobin, or blood nitrogen, calcium and phosphorus concentrations. The electrocardiogram showed no abnormalities which could be attributed to direct action on the heart, and from a few observations made, marihuana appeared to be without effect on gastric motility and secretion. The positive results found, as well as the occurrence of nausea and vomiting, an increase in the frequency of urination, and the sensation of hunger and an increase in appetite, may be considered results of central nervous excitation, producing peripheral effects through the autonomic nervous system.

The psychological study, planned and carried out by experienced psychologists, was concomitant with the general medical one and was devoted to determining the effects of marihuana on psychomotor responses and certain special abilities, on intellectual functioning, and on emotional reactions and personality structure.

For psychomotor effects, procedures were followed which gave records affording quantitative measurement. Static equilibrium and hand steadiness were the functions most strongly affected by marihuana. The body swaying was general in direction and not greater in one axis than in others. These effects came on during the first hour after the extract was given, reached a peak in about four hours, and persisted for some eight hours. After smoking, the effects came on much sooner—within a few minutes—and were of shorter duration, about three hours. Complex hand and foot reactions showed impairment, but simple reaction time, the strength of grip, speed of tapping, auditory acuity and musical ability, and estimation of short time intervals and small linear distances were unchanged.

The findings in the women corresponded to those in the male subjects. In both groups there was marked individual variability, irrespective of dosage.

It was found that marihuana in an effective dose impairs intellectual functioning in general. Included under this heading are adverse effects on speed and accuracy in performance, on the application of acquired knowledge, on carrying out routine tasks, on memory, and on capacity for learning.

Marihuana does not change the basic personality structure of the individual. It lessens inhibition and this brings out what is latent in his thoughts and emotions but it does not evoke responses which would otherwise be totally alien to him. It induces a feeling of self-confidence, but this is expressed in thought rather than in performance. There is, in fact, evidence of a diminution in physical activity. While suggestibility may be increased by small doses, larger ones tend to induce a negativistic attitude.

From the study as a whole, it is concluded that marihuana is not a drug of addiction, comparable to morphine, and that if tolerance is acquired, this is of a very limited degree. Furthermore those who have been smoking marihuana for a period of years showed no mental or physical deterioration which may be attributed to the drug.

The lessening of inhibitions and repression, the euphoric state, the feeling of adequacy, the freer expression of thoughts and ideas, and the increase in appetite for food brought about by marihuana suggest therapeutic possibilities. From limited observations on addicts undergoing morphine withdrawal and on certain types of psychopathic disturbances, the impression was gained that marihuana had beneficial effects, but much more extensive and controlled study is required for definite conclusions to be drawn concerning therapeutic usage. It should be borne in mind that the effects of marihuana, more than in the case of other drugs, are quite variable in different individuals and in the same one at different times.

The chapter on the pharmacology of marihuana, prepared by Dr. Loewe, reviews the results of collaborative work of three laboratories (The Pharmacological Laboratory at the Cornell Medical College, the William Albert Noyes Laboratory at the University of Illinois, and the Laboratory of the Bureau of Narcotics at Washington, D. C.) which led to the discovery of the active principles, the elucidation of their origin, and the assembling of data on the relationship between chemical structure and biological activity. The chapter is introduced by a survey of the geographical distribution and botanical relationships of plants with marihuana activity.

The principles involved in bioassay are discussed and a method for marihuana assay described. The synthetic tetrahydrocannabinol of Adams was taken as the standard of reference and the characteristic reaction of ataxia in dogs measured quantitatively for the degree of activity. By this method the potency of samples and preparations of marihuana and of natural and synthetic principles has been determined and relationships between chemical structure and pharmacological activity elucidated.

The main components which have been isolated from marihuana oil containing the active principles are cannabidiol, cannabinol and isomeric tetrahydrocannabinols. The first two, but not the last, have been obtained as crystalline substances. The chemical structure and synthesis of these compounds have been described by Adams.

The typical effects of marihuana on man are ascribed to actions on the central nervous system. In dogs, the characteristic effect is ataxia. A delayed increase in pulse rate, a decrease in respiratory rate and blood pressure, and retching and vomiting were also observed. These effects are produced by tetrahydrocannabinol but not by cannabinol or cannabidiol. A derivative of the latter, tetrahydrocannabidiol, after a latent period of from thirty to seventy minutes following intravenous injection, had a specific convulsant action on the dog.

In rabbits a characteristic effect of marihuana extracts is corneal areflexia. This is also not produced by cannabidiol or cannabinol but does occur after tetrahydrocannabinol. However, impure oil mixtures have this action to a greater extent, from which it is suggested that a third unknown principle is present in the plant.

Cannabidiol has a synergistic hypnotic action with pernoston in mice. Neither cannabinol nor the synthetic tetrahydrocannabidiols had this effect.

The ataxia action of marihuana was considerably increased by a central stimulant, benzedrine.

No evidence was found of an acquired tolerance for the drug.

In examination of the data presented in the detailed clinical study it is seen that the effects reported were in the main those produced by the extract of marihuana taken by mouth. With the extract, the absorption is gradual and the action persists as long as the active principles are circulating throughout the body. The doses given were fixed ones and once taken the effects were beyond the subjects' control. Giving the extract thus afforded a longer period for study and insured greater accuracy in dosage. In New York, as far as is known, marihuana is rarely if ever taken in this form but is smoked in cigarettes. However, it is shown in the study that the effects from smoking correspond in kind to those from the extract. The difference is that, in smoking, the effects come on promptly and are of much shorter duration. How marked the reaction becomes depends on the number of cigarettes smoked and this is entirely under the subjects' control. The sensations desired are pleasurable ones—a feeling of contentment, inner satisfaction, free play of imagination. Once this stage is reached, the experienced user realizes that with further smoking the pleasurable sensations will be changed to unpleasant ones and so takes care to avoid this.

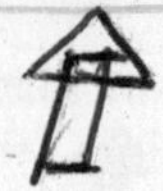